INTENSIVE CORONARY CARE

A Manual For Nurses

LAWRENCE E. MELTZER, M.D.
Director, Section of Clinical Investigation
Director, Coronary Care Unit, Presbyterian-
University of Pennsylvania Medical Center, Philadelphia

ROSE PINNEO, R.N., M.S.
Assistant Professor of Nursing; Clinical Specialist in
Cardiovascular Nursing, University of Rochester, School of
Medicine and Dentistry, Department of Nursing,
Rochester, New York

J. RODERICK KITCHELL, M.D.
Director of Medical Services, Abington Memorial Hospital,
Abington; Assistant Clinical Professor of Medicine, University
of Pennsylvania School of Medicine, Philadelphia

NEW REVISED EDITION

THE CHARLES PRESS *Publishers Inc.*
A Division of the Robert J. Brady Company
Bowie, Maryland 20715

Library of Congress catalog card number: 71-130581

THE CHARLES PRESS *Publishers, Inc.*
Bowie, Maryland 20715

Printed in the United States of America

SIXTH PRINTING

Preface

The concept of intensive coronary care proposed in the original edition of this book has now become an established method of treatment for patients with acute myocardial infarction in hospitals throughout the world. It has been our premise that intensive coronary care is primarily, and above all, a system of specialized nursing care and that its success is predicated almost wholly on the ability of nurses to assume a new and demanding role. It was for this reason that the manual was written for nurses rather than physicians — a deliberate reversal of the customary order for presenting a new medical plan.

Any reluctance of the nursing profession to accept or adopt this system of care would have been quite understandable since the duties and responsibilities assigned to nurses transcended traditional nursing practices and might well have been viewed as awesome. In accepting this challenge and demonstrating remarkable competence as the key members of the coronary care team, nurses have been instrumental in saving the lives of thousands of patients with acute myocardial infarction; in doing so, they have broadly expanded the horizons of clinical nursing and have earned the sincere respect of their physician and nurse colleagues and the gratitude of their patients.

During the past five years the original system of intensive coronary care has been modified in several ways. The emphasis of the program now is focused on the prevention of complications rather than their emergency treatment; in addition, important advances have been made in techniques (e.g., transvenous cardiac pacing) and in drug therapy — all of which have influenced (expanded) the nursing role. The manual has been revised at this time to keep pace with these new developments.

The unprecedented success of the original edition of this manual (more than 300,000 copies in print) has served to restrain us from making any major changes in the style or format of the book. Hopefully, we have preserved the simplicity and clarity that characterized the first version.

As might be anticipated, the research that led to this publication could not have been started, no less accomplished, without the help of certain leaders in the nursing profession who were willing and anxious to see if clinical nursing could be upgraded to the level demanded by the system of intensive coronary care. In this regard we are particularly indebted to Dr. Faye Abdellah, for her unwavering assistance and sound advice. Nor could this undertaking have been attempted without the support of Mr. Carl Mosher, Executive Vice-President, Presbyterian-University of Pennsylvania Medical Center, who recognized the potential value of this plan long before it became a reality. But our greatest debt is to the superb group of nurses who participated in this research effort and helped to develop intensive coronary care to its present state.

Lawrence E. Meltzer, M.D.
Rose Pinneo, R.N., M.S.
J. Roderick Kitchell, M.D.

Philadelphia, Pennsylvania
August 1970

Contents

The Technique of Electrocardioversion and the Nursing Role
The Technique of Emergency Defibrillation

The studies conducted at the Presbyterian-University of Pennsylvania Medical Center, upon which this book is based, were supported by Grants #NU00096, Intensive Nursing Care in Acute Myocardial Infarction and #NU00263, Specialized Nursing Care in Acute Circulatory Failure, from the Research Grants Branch, Division of Nursing, Department of Health, Education and Welfare, U. S. Public Health Service.

CHAPTER 1

Coronary Heart Disease

When the incredible complexity of the human system is considered along with the vast number of possible sources of illness and death, it seems incongruous that the life of so many depends finally on the health of two small arteries; but the fact is undeniable. Disease of the coronary arteries has become the one greatest threat to life and it is responsible for more than 500,000 deaths - or one-third of *all* deaths - in the United States each year.

As the sole blood supply to the heart musculature (the myocardium), the coronary arteries assume extreme importance. Any significant interference with the flow through these vessels can impair the entire function of the myocardium with dire consequences including sudden death.

The basic disease process affecting the coronary arteries is *atherosclerosis:* where fatty materials deposit as plaques, along the inner lining (intima) of these vessels and narrow the passage. If the arterial obstruction reaches a point where the blood supply becomes insufficient to meet the demands of the myocardium then coronary heart disease (CHD) is said to exist.

The reason that coronary heart disease is the number one cause of death in this country is readily apparent: the cause of atherosclerosis is still unknown, there is no proven way to halt its progression once it becomes manifest and finally there are no diagnostic means presently available to detect coronary artery disease until it is far advanced.

An unrelenting search has been in progress for more than 50 years attempting to ascertain why and how the coronary arteries are affected by atherosclerosis. Although no specific cause for coronary atherosclerosis has been found thus far, several theories have been proposed to explain the disease.

At first it was thought that coronary atherosclerosis was simply related to aging and that the deposition of plaques within the arteries was, in effect, a degenerative process. It became clear that this concept was not correct since coronary heart disease was observed with increasing frequency among relatively young people.

Because the plaques within the coronary arteries were found to contain fatty substances (particularly cholesterol), the major direction of subsequent research was aimed at seeking a causal relationship between intake of dietary fats and the development of

1

coronary heart disease. There is now good reason to believe that this premise has validity. Several epidemiologic studies have shown that the incidence of premature coronary heart disease (that is, coronary disease developing before the age of 60) can be related to the different dietary patterns of various societies. Specifically, affluent countries as the U.S.A. where animal fats constitute a large percentage of the total diet, have a very high rate of CHD and poorer countries where animal fat intake is much less, have a low incidence of the disease. This gross disparity in animal fat intake (e.g., butter, eggs, milk, etc.) between these societies is believed to account for the fact that "normal" serum cholesterol levels in the U.S.A. may be 200-250 mg. %, whereas in those countries in which CHD is infrequent the comparable cholesterol levels are only 100-150 mg. %. Further evidence in support of this argument is the reported decrease in deaths due to CHD during World War II in those countries where animal fats became scarce, followed by a prompt increase in the death rate once the economy improved and fats were again available after the war ended. From data of this type it has been concluded by many that overeating (particularly of fatty foods) is a prime factor in the etiology of coronary heart disease.

Although most observers seem to agree with the concept that gluttony is associated with CHD, considerable doubt has been expressed that this one factor itself can fully account for the vast difference in the incidence of the disease in various countries. It has been suggested that other influences are of equal, or perhaps greater, importance in explaining this variation. One alternative hypothesis would relate the incidence of CHD to stresses of our civilization. In some unexplained manner emotional tensions are thought to induce certain biochemical or physical changes which ultimately result in atherosclerosis. Presumably, on this basis, highly-competitive, aggressive societies have a high rate of CHD while in primitive, less-demanding countries (e.g., Africa) the disease is uncommon. In other words, CHD is considered by some to be a disease of "over-civilization."

It should be recognized that both of these etiological theories have not been proven specifically but are founded on what many still consider as circumstantial evidence. (Facetiously, it would be possible to correlate these same epidemiologic findings with other cincumstantial data, including the number of automobiles, television sets, or bathtubs in the respective populations).

While the true cause of coronary atherosclerosis remains unknown, there are nevertheless a few substantial leads which ultimately may identify the underlying basis of the disease. The most promising clues are as follows:

    a)   coronary heart disease is distinctly more prevalent in men than in women during the child-bearing age. After the menopause, however, the incidence of CHD in females rises rapidly and equals the male rate thereafter. This pattern is quite unlike that of men where gross evidence of coronary atherosclerosis may be found at young (18-25) ages. This age-sex discrepancy suggests that a hormonal influence may be important in the disease.

b) patients with diabetes, regardless of the degree of control, have at least a four-fold increase in the incidence of CHD, compared to non-diabetics. This unquestionable finding, along with data showing that other metabolic diseases (e.g., gout) also are associated with a high incidence of CHD, suggests that a biochemical disturbance may be central to the disease process.

c) coronary atherosclerosis appears to be influenced by heredity and a familial pattern of the disease has long been recognized.

Disappointingly, none of these leads have, as yet, provided an answer to coronary disease and perhaps the most valuable approach to the problem at the present time involves an attempt to identify certain factors which seem to influence the development of CHD.

It has been shown that a high percentage (but not all) of patients with CHD have many characteristics in common. These characteristics are described as "risk factors" and include the following:

a) a family history of CHD
b) hypertension
c) high serum cholesterol
d) gout
e) diabetes
f) overweight
g) cigarette smoking
h) muscular body build with heavy bones (mesomorph)
i) sedentary existence
j) aggressive, competitive personality.

There is no definite evidence that any of these risk factors actually *cause* CHD but it appears that patients who have a large number of these conditions are high-risk candidates for CHD and conversely the absence of these risk factors predicts little likelihood of developing the disease. For example, an overweight man with diabetes and hypertension who smokes cigarettes and leads a sedentary life has an enormously greater chance of sustaining a heart attack than a person without any of these characteristics.

THE COURSE OF CORONARY HEART DISEASE

Once atherosclerosis has developed within the coronary arteries the disease may take several different courses:

1) **Unrecognized Coronary Heart Disease**

   If the degree of arterial obstruction is minimal and does not significantly reduce the blood supply to the myocardium then the disease may very well be unsuspected by the patient or his physician. Results of autopsy studies from patients dying of other causes indicate that this is a frequent situation. In fact, it appears that most men in the United States have some evidence of coronary atherosclerosis; only the degree of involvement varies.

2) **Asymptomatic Coronary Disease**

   Even if the coronary arteries are grossly narrowed by intimal plaques it still does not follow that CHD will be clinically evident and produce symptoms. There is evidence that as gradual occlusion of the coronary arteries takes place, small branches of these arteries may enlarge, or new vessels may form to help bring more blood to the myocardium. This additional blood supply, called *collateral circulation* is of great importance in determining the clinical course since this network of vessels is often substantial enough to maintain adequate flow to the myocardium despite gross atherosclerosis. It is the *total* blood supply to the myocardium, rather than the state of the two main coronary arteries that determines whether or not the disease will be symptomatic.

3) **Symptomatic Coronary Heart Disease (Angina Pectoris)**

   In the event that the total blood supply is inadequate to meet the demands of the myocardium, overt, symptomatic coronary heart disease exists. The classical indication of this impaired circulation to the myocardium is the presence of a distinctive type of chest pain called *angina pectoris*. As a result of the compromised blood supply the amount of oxygen available to the myocardium is reduced; it is this insufficient oxygenation *(ischemia)* that causes angina pectoris. In other words, angina pectoris represents a warning signal indicating that the myocardium does not have a sufficient amount of oxygen to meet its demand at the moment. Because this one symptom is often the entire key to the diagnosis of CHD it is extremely important that the clinical pattern of angina be fully understood:

Site of pain. The chest pain reflecting myocardial ischemia is located most often directly under the breast bone. It may radiate from this *substernal* location to either the left or right arm, the neck, the jaw, the teeth, or to the upper back. In some instances, the pain occurs only at these latter sites without a substernal component. This pattern is much less common than pure substernal pain.

Type and quality of pain. The pain is usually described as a pressure, or tightness within the chest. Some patients clench their fists over the chest in describing the sensation. Anginal pain is *steady* and is not influenced by movement of the body, by breathing, or breath-holding. This constancy of substernal pain is the most typical aspect of angina and is more important than other descriptive qualities (e.g., constriction, pressure, indigestion, etc.)

Occurrence of pain. Any circumstance that increases the myocardial need for oxygen is capable of producing angina. In general, oxygen demand is dependent on the amount of work the heart performs. As would be anticipated on this basis, angina is most commonly noted with physical exertion where the heart rate and work (and in turn, oxygen requirements) are increased. Conversely, when the activity stops, the oxygen demand falls promptly and the pain subsides. This relationship - activity, pain, rest, disappearance of pain - is typical of myocardial ischemia and distinguishes angina from other non-ischemic causes of chest pain where this pattern does not exist. In addition to exertion, sudden emotional outbursts (anger, fear, the excitement of watching a football game, etc.) or the appearance of rapid heart rates frequently cause angina; these states increase the work of the heart and its need for oxygen. In some patients angina occurs during sleep or at rest in a paradoxical fashion for reasons not wholly understood; dreams have been incriminated.

Duration of pain. Angina is characteristically of *short* duration, lasting only seconds to a minute before abating with rest. The cessation of pain indicates that the myocardial demand for oxygen has been met, and that the oxygen deficit was only transient and non-destructive to the tissues.

Relief of pain. Another distinctive feature of angina is the prompt relief of pain that follows the use of nitroglycerin. Failure of nitroglycerin, administered sublingually, to terminate ischemic chest pain promptly is unusual and is cause for suspicion that the pain is not anginal in origin. Nitroglycerin is thought to dilate the coronary vessels thus increasing the blood flow and oxygen supply to the myocardium.

4) Coronary Insufficiency

In some patients, either as a gradual change in an existing anginal pattern, or as an initial symptom, the chest pain does not stop promptly with rest or nitroglycerin but continues for 5 to 10 minutes or longer. This persistance of pain implies that ischemia has prevailed all along. This type of prolonged angina is described as *coronary insufficiency* (an unfortunate term since obviously all forms of angina are due to coronary insufficiency) in contrast to either the short-lived pain of angina pectoris or, at the other extreme, the unrelenting, severe pain associated with the complete ischemia of *myocardial infarction*. This "intermediate" type of angina is often an ominous symptom, being a frequent forerunner of complete coronary occlusion. For this reason, many prefer to call this form of pain *pre-infarction angina*. Theoretically, coronary insufficiency suggests that adequate oxygenation was restored before actual destruction of the myocardium occurred; however, it is often impossible to rule out the likelihood that small areas of muscle necrosis resulted from oxygen deprivation during the episode of pain.

5) Myocardial Infarction

If the insufficiency of blood and oxygen to a portion of the myocardium is profound and sustained, the involved cells cannot survive, and *local* death (necrosis) occurs in this area. This destructive state is termed *acute myocardial infarction*. The event which produced the infarction is often called a coronary thrombosis, a coronary occlusion, a coronary, or a heart attack. These latter terms are used synonymously in clinical practice to describe what properly should be called an acute myocardial infarction. Nearly all instances of acute myocardial infarction are due to atherosclerosis involving the coronary arteries. Very rarely can the arteries be narrowed by other processes including syphilis, collagen diseases, or emboli from other sites.

The final insult from coronary atherosclerosis is usually the actual obstruction of a main coronary artery or its branches; in most cases, this occlusion occurs *suddenly*. The exact reason that a coronary vessel blocks off at a certain moment is not completely understood, but three different causes have been incriminated: 1) a blood clot may develop on the rough surface of the atherosclerotic plaque and occlude the lumen of the artery (coronary thrombosis); 2) the atherosclerotic lesion may irritate the underlying arterial wall and cause bleeding beneath the plaque; this sub-intimal hemorrhage dislodges the plaque which then obstructs the vessel; and 3) a piece of a large plaque may break off and block a smaller artery. While these mechanisms offer a logical explanation for this sudden event, it is now clear that neither clot formation nor plaque disruption can account for *all* myocardial infarctions. Autopsy studies have shown that myocardial infarction may occur despite the fact that the arteries are still patent and not completely closed. In these latter instances, it is presumed that at a particular time the heart may have an enormous demand for oxygen (e.g., during sudden vigorous physical exertion, as shoveling snow) which cannot be met by the available blood supply. In effect, even though the arteries are not completely obstructed, the demand for oxygen simply overwhelms its supply and tissue necrosis occurs because of this relative deprivation. A similar situation may result from profound anemia (e.g., gastro-intestinal hemorrhage) where oxygen available to the myocardium is grossly reduced and infarction may take place in the presence of patent arteries.

Once the coronary circulation is interrupted and myocardial infarction results, a series of events follow which place life and death in balance. This book concerns itself with these events and describes a new concept of specialized care (*Intensive Coronary Care*) designed to lower the death rate once myocardial infarction has occurred.

CHAPTER 2

Acute Myocardial Infarction

THE PATIENT'S HISTORY

Most patients with acute myocardial infarction seek medical assistance because of *chest pain*. The pain is usually quite distinctive; it occurs suddenly and is of severe, crushing quality. It is more intense than the pain of angina or coronary insufficiency and may be unlike any sensation the patient has previously experienced. Typically, the pain is concentrated directly beneath the sternum but it frequently radiates across the chest or to the arms and neck. Patients commonly describe the pain as a heavy weight or pressure or a knot in the chest.

The pain does not necessarily occur with exertion as does angina; in fact, it frequently begins during sleep. Its occurrence after eating explains why many patients interpret the pain as indigestion.

The chest pain is *continuous* and is not relieved by change in body position, breath-holding or by home remedies (e.g., bicarbonate) that the patient may try.

Shortly after the onset of the substernal pain drenching perspiration usually begins and nausea and vomiting often occur at this time. Fear and apprehension are usual and most patients sense that a catastrophe has happened. Within minutes, many patients are aware of dyspnea and marked weakness. This symptom complex of substernal pain, sweating, nausea, vomiting along with dyspnea and weakness can be considered the typical history of acute myocardial infarction.

Not all patients present such typical histories; there are many variants of the story. Sometimes the major pain is not in the chest but, as with angina, is located in the neck, the arms or the jaws. Sweating, nausea, vomiting and dyspnea may not accompany this referred pain. On other occasions, pain may be absent and myocardial infarction is suspected because the patient has collapsed suddenly, usually without warning.

Acute myocardial infarction may also develop during surgery. In this situation, the symptoms are masked by anesthesia and the diagnosis of infarction is considered because of an unexplained drop in blood pressure or the development of shock during a surgical procedure.

A few patients presumably sustain acute myocardial infarction without any chest pain or other symptoms. This diagnosis is surmised when there is evidence of an *old* infarction on a routine electrocardiogram and yet the patient denies any previous symptoms; these are called *silent* infarctions.

Lastly, some patients develop serious complications of acute myocardial infarction immediately after the occlusion and in these instances it is the complication itself (e.g., sudden left ventricular failure or an arrhythmia) that causes suspicion that an infarction has occurred.

THE CLINICAL COURSE IMMEDIATELY AFTER INFARCTION

It is quite apparent that the heart may respond in several different ways to the abrupt interruption of its blood supply; some patients develop serious or lethal complications almost instantly, while others never experience any difficulties. It is not known with certainty which factors actually influence the heart's behavior once coronary occlusion has occurred. It has been presumed that the size of the infarction is the most important determinant of the subsequent clinical course. In general, if a main artery is occluded and there is extensive myocardial damage the course and prognosis are thought to be much poorer than if a branch vessel is blocked and the resultant injury is small. This relationship however is not constant and many patients with limited areas of tissue destruction develop serious complications. Because of this disparity it is evident that other factors play a role in determining the outcome of the illness. Considered to be of particular importance in this regard is the degree of collateral blood supply that can instantly be diverted to the deprived area of the myocardium. If an extensive collateral supply exists the original insult to the tissues may be minimized and, conversely, if there are only few blood vessels in the surrounding area, oxygenation of the myocardium cannot be enhanced. Because of these variants (along with probably other influences which are not well understood) several possible clinical pictures may occur with acute myocardial infarction:

1) If the infarcted area is limited in size, and enough blood is diverted to the site by collateral channels, the myocardium may continue to function quite normally. The heart's pumping action may not be affected and the rate and rhythm of the heart are not necessarily disturbed. The pain gradually subsides in these instances and the patient appears in no distress.

2) When the involved area is larger and if there is only trivial collateral assistance, the myocardium may become sufficiently embarrassed so that its function is impaired. This may be manifested by signs of decreased pumping action of the heart (heart failure) or by disturbances in the rate and rhythm of the heart beat (arrhythmias). The degree of impairment may vary greatly; some patients have only mild shortness of breath and

minor arrhythmias while others are critically ill with marked dyspnea, pulmonary edema and life-threatening arrhythmias.

3) If the pumping action of the heart is grossly reduced as a result of extensive structural damage to the myocardium, the left ventricle is simply unable to pump sufficient blood throughout the body to sustain circulation to the vital organs. On this basis the blood pressure falls, the heart rate increases, the urinary output decreases and skin becomes cold and clammy. This state is called *cardiogenic shock;* most patients with this complication die within hours.

4) In some patients death occurs almost instantly after occlusion has occurred. These *sudden* deaths are almost always the result of lethal *arrhythmias* resulting from extraordinary changes in the electrical activity of the heart. In these instances the heart either stops abruptly (ventricular standstill) or beats ineffectively in a mere quivering fashion (ventricular fibrillation). There is no clear relationship between the size of the infarction and the occurrence of sudden, arrhythmic deaths. Studies have shown that probably 50% of *all* deaths from acute myocardial infarction occur within the first hour after the attack.

Because of these different possibilities it can be appreciated that some patients admitted to the hospital with acute myocardial infarction may have no pain by the time they arrive and are not in distress while others are near death from cardiogenic shock or acute heart failure when first seen. The ultimate clinical course is related to a large degree, but certainly *not* entirely, to the admission picture. *Complications can develop at any time in any patient.*

THE PHYSICAL EXAMINATION

When the physician examines the patient he attempts fundamentally to ascertain whether or not complications of the infarction have developed. First of all, he seeks signs of circulatory failure as evidenced by the presence of rales at the bases of the lungs, distended neck veins and a gallop rhythm (among other findings). He is also concerned about the possibility of cardiogenic shock and determines the patient's blood pressure, pulse rate, urinary output, and other physical signs of this complication. In addition to this phase of the examination, the physician observes the rate and rhythm of the heart to identify arrhythmic disturbances.

It is understandable that the physical examination may be quite normal in those patients where the circulation has not been impaired and in whom arrhythmias have not developed. Furthermore, it should be realized that acute myocardial infarction cannot be distinguished from other forms of heart disease (which also may produce arrhythmias and circulatory failure) solely by physical examination. In this sense, the physical examination is more important in assessing the complications of myocardial infarction than in its diagnosis.

THE DIAGNOSIS OF ACUTE MYOCARDIAL INFARCTION

The diagnosis of acute myocardial infarction is made essentially in three steps:

1) **The Patient's History**

In many ways the patient's story of his illness is the prime factor in reaching the diagnosis of acute myocardial infarction. It is because of the history that the physician *suspects* the diagnosis and admits the patient to the hospital. The development of severe, substernal pain associated with nausea, sweating, and the other features already mentioned is often so distinctive that the physician can safely anticipate subsequent confirmation of his diagnosis by the electrocardiogram and enzyme studies. However, the history, regardless of how typical it may be, is not diagnostic in its own right and other steps must be taken to prove that acute infarction has actually occurred.

2) **The Electrocardiogram**

The diagnosis of acute myocardial infarction can only be made *definitively* by electrocardiographic means. When injury and local death (infarction) of myocardial tissue occurs, characteristic findings reflecting these changes are found in the electrocardiographic tracing. On many occasions, the initial diagnostic (12 lead) electrocardiogram fails to show definite evidence of an infarction and subsequent (serial) tracings must be made over the next several days until definite electrocardiographic proof has evolved.

It is important to realize that the electrocardiogram does not show the actual extent of damage and, by itself, is not a true index of the seriousness of the attack. The diagnosis of acute infarction cannot, and should not, be made unless characteristic electrocardiographic changes are finally demonstrated.

3) Enzyme Studies

In some instances, where the patient may give an impressive history suggesting acute myocardial infarction, but where the electrocardiograms show equivocal, (rather than definite) changes, other studies are necessary to verify the diagnosis. The most important of these laboratory determinations involves the measurement of certain enzymes in the blood. The basis of these tests is as follows: several enzymes normally reside within the cells comprising the myocardium; when the myocardium is injured these enzymes escape into the blood stream where they can be detected and measured. Thus, after acute myocardial infarction a characteristic elevation of these substances in the serum is to be expected.

The three most useful enzyme studies used to confirm the diagnosis of acute myocardial infarction are:

Creatine Phosphokinase (CPK)

This enzyme is the first to rise after infarction and elevated levels can be detected within 6 hours. After 2-3 days, the CPK levels usually return to normal. For this reason the determination should be performed at the time of admission and repeated in 24 and 48 hours.

Serum Glutamic Oxaloacetic Transaminase (SGOT)

SGOT levels rise less rapidly than CPK after infarction. Typical increases are usually noted after 24 hours and persist for 3-4 days. Therefore, the concentrations of this enzyme should be measured at 24, 48 and 72 hours after the attack. While SGOT levels are generally reliable in confirming myocardial damage it should be recognized that this particular enzyme can also be elevated from other sources, especially liver diseases.

Lactic Dehydrogenase (LDH)

The serum levels of LDH increase at a slower rate than CPK or SGOT following infarction. Significant elevations do not usually occur until the second or third day and they last for 5-6 days. Accordingly, this determination should be performed on days 3,4 and 5 after the attack if the other enzyme levels have not solved the problem.

It should be fully appreciated that the diagnosis of acute myocardial infarction must never be *solely* on the basis of these enzyme studies; the value of these tests is only supplemental. Conversely, negative results of these studies should not be grounds to abandon the diagnosis of myocardial infarction in the presence of a typical history and characteristic electrocardiographic findings.

THE COURSE DURING HOSPITALIZATION

In general, the clinical course after infarction can be considered in two phases: the *acute* phase, which usually involves the first 5 days following the attack, and the *subacute* phase which concerns the remaining period of hospitalization. During the acute phase patients are treated in an intensive coronary care unit.

The most characteristic aspect of the acute phase of myocardial infarction is its *uncertainty;* there is no typical course. The variation in the clinical picture is quite remarkable but three broad patterns exist:

1) There are some patients whose course is truly uncomplicated. They show no evidence of cardiogenic shock, acute heart failure, arrhythmias, or other problems during this usually critical period of the illness. Most of these patients make uneventful recoveries regardless of the type of treatment employed. As will be shown subsequently such uncomplicated courses are much less frequent than those with complications.

2) Among other patients the illness appears benign at the time of admission but suddenly major complications develop. These complications account for nearly all of the deaths and it is the unpredictability of these catastrophes that makes myocardial infarction such a lethal disease. The concept of intensive coronary care is based on the immediate detection and treatment of these complications. By its ability to prevent sudden unexpected death in this group of patients the system of intensive coronary care has made its greatest contribution.

3) When complications already exist at the time of admission, the clinical course is usually hectic and the prognosis becomes extremely poor. For example, if shock is present when the patient is first seen there is a 90 % likelihood that the patient will die within the next 48 hours and if acute heart failure is evident on admission, the mortality may be as high as 50%. Therefore, the original clinical picture is very important in determining the ultimate course of the attack; but an uncomplicated picture on admission should not lead to a false sense of security for reasons stated in the preceding paragraphs.

That acute myocardial infarction may have such widely divergent

14

courses explains why the death rate may be 90% at one extreme and zero to 5% at the other. Probably no other disease behaves in this unpredictable fashion. The final outcome of the illness depends on the presence or absence of complications.

THE COMPLICATIONS OF ACUTE MYOCARDIAL INFARCTION

There are five major complications that threaten life after acute myocardial infarction.*

1) **Arrhythmias**

Disturbances in the cardiac rate and rhythm (arrhythmias) are the most common complications of acute myocardial infarction. Their presence poses two serious threats. Arrhythmias may produce sudden death and secondly they reduce the pumping efficiency of the myocardium, leading to acute heart failure. Probably 80%, or more, of patients with acute infarction have some disturbance of rate and rhythm during the acute phase of the illness. *Arrhythmias can occur at any time without warning.*

2) **Acute Heart Failure**

The contractile ability of the myocardium is often reduced following infarction causing the heart to fail as a pumping system. Such failure can occur suddenly resulting in acute pulmonary edema, or gradually, if the ventricle recovers from the original ischemia but falters subsequently. In these latter instances, there may be early findings to suggest impending heart failure. Clinical signs of heart failure are observed in about 60% of patients; the degree of this pumping deficit varies considerably.

3) **Cardiogenic Shock**

When the heart is unable to sustain enough circulation to provide adequate oxygen to the vital organs and tissues cardiogenic shock is said to exist. This is by far the most serious complication of acute myocardial infarction; the mortality is at least 80% with current methods of therapy. Cardiogenic shock occurs more frequently within the first several hours after the attack but can develop at any time.

* These complications, including their diagnosis and treatment, form the basis for intensive coronary care and are considered in appropriate detail in subsequent chapters. They are mentioned here to allow an uninterrupted picture of the disease.

4) Thrombo-embolism

There is a propensity for blood to clot on the inner wall of the injured left ventricle. These clots may break loose and leave the heart (as emboli) and block the arterial supply to the brain, abdomen, or extremities. Emboli of this type are less frequent than those arising from the deep veins of the legs (presumably due to stasis of blood) which eventually find their way to the lungs and produce pulmonary infarction. Embolic phenomena, either from the left ventricle, or from the leg veins, can produce sudden death but this complication is not common and accounts for a small percentage of all deaths.

5) Rupture of the Left Ventricle

When there is extensive damage to the ventricular wall the necrotic area may weaken leading to a rupture of the ventricle. When this catastrophe occurs blood from the ventricle instantly fills the surrounding pericardial sac and causes compression of heart (cardiac tamponade). Death follows, usually within minutes. Ventricular rupture develops most often 7-10 days after the original infarction but this relationship is not absolute. Along with thrombo-embolism, ventricular ruptures constitute only a small percentage of the total mortality from acute myocardial infarction.

OTHER ASPECTS OF THE ACUTE PHASE

1) Most patients with acute myocardial infarction develop temperature elevations during the acute phase of the illness. Typically, the body temperature rises after the first 24 hours to levels of 100-101 degrees or more and remains elevated for 2-3 days before declining gradually. By the fifth day after the attack the temperature is usually normal. It is thought that this febrile pattern reflects the destruction of myocardial tissue. The white blood count and sedimentation rate also increase during this period for similar reasons.

2) Profound emotional reactions are often noted among patients with acute myocardial infarction within several days after the attack. The basis of this response is readily understandable in most instances: the abrupt interruption of normal life, the fear of death and the possibility of permanent invalidism are strong psychological threats. Because the patient's response (behavior) to this stress is influenced by numerous factors inherent in his personality the spectrum of reactions is very wide.

THE SUBACUTE PHASE OF MYOCARDIAL INFARCTION

The incidence of complications lessens markedly after the first five days and for this reason patients are usually transferred from the coronary care unit to other facilities within the hospital at this time.

During this remaining period of hospitalization (the sub-acute phase) the infarcted area begins to heal. In the absence of serious complications the total hospital stay is about three weeks in duration (which includes the period of intensive coronary care). During this time physical activity is restricted in order to limit the work of the heart as it heals. Some physicians prefer to keep patients at complete bed rest in this interim. However, there has been a gradual tendency to liberalize certain physical activity in the subacute phase and to allow patients to use bathroom facilities and to sit in arm chairs. The use of chair rest, rather than bed rest, is considered beneficial not only for the emotional support that is derived from being out of bed but also because the sitting position may actually be more effective in terms of circulatory efficiency.

In *uncomplicated* cases few medications are necessary during the subacute phase. Anticoagulant therapy is commonly continued through this period (to prevent thromboembolism) and while the pertinent evidence seems to support this practice there is still considerable controversy about the true value of anticoagulation and some physicians do not use anticoagulants. The hospital course of patients who experience complications varies with the nature of the problems and their response to treatment. Understandably the period of hospitalization may be prolonged if serious complications develop.

While the subacute phase is undoubtedly less hazardous than the acute phase, substantial evidence has accumulated to indicate that the period after transfer from the coronary care unit is by no means without danger. *Complications can develop at any time during the hospital stay.*

THE PERIOD AFTER HOSPITALIZATION (CONVALESCENT PHASE)

Following discharge from the hospital it is customary for patients to remain at home on limited activity until healing of the myocardium has occurred. In general, necrotic areas heal within 6-8 weeks after the attack. This implies that if a patient was hospitalized for 3-4 weeks the period of convalescence at home will be an additional 3-4 weeks. The length of convalescence varies primarily with the patient's age and the functional capacity of his heart after the infarction.

While at home, physical activity is gradually increased. Bed rest is usually unnecessary but stair climbing or household chores should be minimized. After the healing phase has ended a deliberate program of physical activity is started in order to develop a collateral circulation to the myocardium. It is believed that regulated exercise is of distinct value for this purpose. In a sense, such exercise helps to create what is, in effect, a new blood supply to replace the previously occluded artery. Walking is considered to be an excellent exercise for this purpose, and should be encouraged with the distance increased daily. In addition to its beneficial effect on the heart and circulation, physical activity at this stage is of great value in combatting the weakness and fatigue (so common after an infarction) which result from prolonged disuse of the skeletal muscles.

Most patients, particularly those with uncomplicated courses are able to resume their customary lives (e.g., return to work) about three months after the original attack. These time relationships cannot be rigid and vary from patient to patient according to age, general health, and cardiac reserve. It is increasingly clear that the resumption of a normal life is beneficial and every effort should be made to accomplish this. There is no reason to believe that deliberate inactivity or retiring from work after a myocardial infarction are conducive to longevity; in fact, the evidence is strictly to the contrary.

THE POST-INFARCTION PERIOD

A majority of patients who survive acute myocardial infarction are able to resume normal productive lives. The two major threats to their existence are recurrent myocardial infarction and the development of chronic heart failure (because of residual myocardial weakness).

At the present time there is no sure definite way to protect against these problems but certain practices have evolved which are believed to be beneficial. These include:

1) the control of obesity and the maintenance of normal weight.
2) the treatment of hypertension (if it exists) with the aim of achieving normal blood pressure.
3) a regular and sensible exercise program designed to increase collateral circulation and improve the efficiency of the heart.
4) abstinence from cigarette smoking.
5) control of serum cholesterol (and other lipids) by means of diet or drug therapy.
6) establishing a new way of life to avoid intense competitive goals and seeking emotional tranquillity.

Life expectancy after a myocardial infarction cannot be clearly defined for the individual patient because of the multiplicity of factors that influence survival. But if *all* patients are considered (regardless of age) available statistics suggest that 50% will survive at least five years and 25% will be alive after ten years. These rates are deceptive for younger patients where longevity may be considerably greater.

CHAPTER 3

The System of Intensive Coronary Care

THE PROBLEM OF CORONARY HEART DISEASE (CHD)

A way to halt the mounting death rate from CHD is urgently needed. As noted, during the last year in the United States more than 500,000 people, a high percentage of whom were in the most productive years of life, died from this one cause. The enormity of this fatality rate is brought into perspective by noting that all forms of cancer together caused less than half this number (250,000) of deaths.

Until now the major attack against the disease has been an unwavering search for the cause of atherosclerosis with the underlying hope that once the source was identified it would prove to be preventable, or at least, reversible. After several decades of research centered on this one approach the problem is still unsolved, and it is becoming increasingly clear that a usable answer will not be forthcoming in the near future. As pointed out in Chapter 1, while certain risk factors for coronary atherosclerosis have been identified (e.g., high cholesterol levels, diabetes, overweight, smoking, hypertension, among others), there is no certainty that any of these factors specifically *cause* atherosclerosis or, more significantly, that by controlling these risks coronary heart disease can be prevented. Present indications are that it will take many more years to fully unravel this complex process and reach a point where coronary atherosclerosis can possibly be prevented or reversed. (Those who believe CHD is an effect of affluent societies might have an even more pessimistic view, since the likelihood of reducing man's present way of life is difficult to imagine.)

If we must accept the conclusion that coronary atherosclerosis is not preventable or reversible at the present time, what else can be done to lower the death rate from CHD?

One suggestion has been the use of surgical techniques to increase the myocardial blood supply once the coronary arteries have become diseased. Methods have been conceived to bring additional blood to the heart by diverting other arteries into the myocardium (revascularization procedures), or by directly removing atherosclerotic plaques from the coronary vessels (endarterectomy). While these methods have been used successfully in some centers, their acceptance overall is still limited. Were these operations to prove wholly successful they would nevertheless have limited application in terms of the vastness of the problem of CHD throughout the world.

A second possibility of combatting CHD concerns the prevention of clot formation on atherosclerotic plaques. Realizing that extensive atherosclerosis may be present for many years in a given patient without ever producing trouble, it has been theorized that unless a clot developed to obstruct the artery, the patient might have continued with an uncomplicated course. The basic question is why does a clot form on one particular day rather than 2 months earlier or a year later? Some research studies suggest that clot formation within arteries may be related to an increase in adhesiveness of blood platelets. Because of this unusual "stickiness," platelets tend to clump together and form the framework of a clot. It has been proposed that platelet adhesiveness may be influenced by certain dietary factors, or perhaps, by the secretion of adrenal hormones (catecholamines). If this premise were correct, it might be possible to prevent clot formation by drug therapy. Although atherosclerosis itself would be unaffected by this approach, the final result of arterial obstruction might be avoided and acute myocardial infarction prevented. Much remains to be learned about this interesting concept.

Perhaps the most meaningful attack against coronary heart disease in the future will involve *primary* prevention of the disease. This implies that deliberate control will have to be exerted against known risk factors beginning in childhood and continued throughout life. Specifically, forthcoming generations would have to recognize dangers such as lack of exercise, gluttony, and smoking, and alter their patterns of living to avoid these risks. This approach will hopefully be more effective than the current plan of *secondary* prevention which attempts to correct these habits (risk factors) long after they have become established. It remains to be seen if future generations will heed this advice.

ANOTHER APPROACH TO THE PROBLEM

Despite the current inability to prevent or reverse coronary atherosclerosis, there is still one possibility for reducing the extraordinary death rate from coronary heart disease: to improve the method of treatment *after* acute myocardial infarction has occurred and to salvage more patients in this way. *At the present time, with customary treatment, about 30% of all patients admitted to hospitals with acute myocardial infarction die during the period of hospitalization.* Recognizing that there are approximately 600,000 patients with acute myocardial infarction admitted to hospitals in this country each year, it is readily apparent that any reduction in hospital mortality that could be achieved would have a significant cumulative effect in combatting the overall death rate from coronary heart disease. For example, if the number of deaths occurring in hospitals could be reduced from 30% to 15%, then as many as 90,000 lives could be saved each year. *The concept of intensive coronary care is based on this premise.* Unlike other proposals for attacking coronary heart disease, this method is both feasible and applicable at the present time.

THE CONCEPT OF INTENSIVE CORONARY CARE

If the hospital mortality rate is to be reduced, it is important to understand why patients die from acute myocardial infarction. It is obvious that occlusion of the coronary artery itself need not be fatal since a majority of patients are able to survive the original insult. *Death results from complications of the occlusion in all instances.* By controlling these complications it is possible to prevent death in many patients.

Although it was known for many years that there were five complications which caused death from acute myocardial infarction, the relative frequency of these catastrophes was not recognized specifically until 1961 when a study involving 761 male patients with acute myocardial infarction (Meltzer, Kitchell, et al) defined the problem. The causes of death among the 171 patients in the study who died were as follows:

Rupture of ventricle	2%
Emboli	8%
Circulatory failure	43%
(Shock and congestive failure)	
Arrhythmias	47%

These data were extremely important in pointing out a way toward improving the survival rate after acute myocardial infarction. It was evident that rupture of the ventricle, the only (practically) untreatable cause of death, was infrequent. Eight percent (8%) of all deaths in this series were due to emboli. (This low percentage was thought to reflect the widespread use of anticoagulant therapy; without such treatment embolic deaths might have been more frequent). Shock and congestive heart failure, representing the inability of the heart to pump effectively, comprised 43% of the fatalities. *The most important observation was the unusually high percentage (47%) of deaths due to arrhythmias.* While sudden and unanticipated deaths resulting from electrical disturbances within the heart (arrhythmias) were not unfamiliar events, their actual frequency in the past had been grossly underestimated. This one finding that nearly one-half of all deaths resulted from arrhythmias became the cornerstone for the concept for intensive coronary care since it was known that *arrhythmic deaths were preventable!*

In fact, it had been shown more than 50 years previously that *ventricular fibrillation,* the arrhythmia responsible for at least 80% of all *sudden deaths,* could be terminated, and life saved, if a powerful electric shock was delivered to the heart immediately after the onset of the arrhythmia. It was believed, originally, that the electrodes (which delivered the electrical shock) had to be applied directly to the surface of the heart. Because this procedure required the chest to be opened (thoracotomy) to expose the heart, the application of this measure was limited primarily to operating rooms.

However, in 1956, Dr. Paul Zoll and his colleagues showed the same life-saving effect (defibrillation) could be achieved with an electric shock administered *externally,* through the intact chest wall. Even this major medical advance had limited practical value until the concept of intensive coronary care was developed because of the extraordinarily short interval – *about 1-2 minutes* – between the onset of ventricular fibrillation and death. The chance of accomplishing this maneuver within such a brief period is understandably remote under normal hospital circumstances. Specifically, successful defibrillation requires that a physician or nurse be present when the arrhythmia begins, that an electrocardiographic machine be brought to the bedside to identify the arrhythmia, and that defibrillation be accomplished – *all within 2 precious minutes or less.* From the results of the previously described study, it is evident that these fortuitous circumstances do not often happen, since arrhythmic deaths occurred with great frequency (47%) despite the availability of trained personnel and necessary equipment in the involved hospitals.

Ventricular standstill, the second of the arrhythmias that cause sudden death is similarly preventable. There was good evidence that if the heartbeat had stopped under some circumstances, it could be reactivated by a regular, intermittent electrical stimulus delivered to the myocardium by a device called a pacemaker. But again, while pacing techniques had been known for more than a dozen years only few lives were saved with this clever method because of the same time limitation: restoration of the heartbeat after ventricular standstill can only be accomplished if the pacemaker is used within 1-2 minutes after the onset of the lethal arrhythmia.

From these facts if follows that if the cardiac rhythm could be observed *continuously* by electronic means and if resuscitative equipment was in constant readiness at the bedside, potentially fatal arrhythmias could be instantly detected and treated; in this way, arrhythmic deaths could be prevented. *Were this scheme successful the total mortality from acute myocardial infarction could possibly be reduced by almost 50%.*

The development of monitoring equipment, which permitted constant surveillance of the cardiac rhythm brought this approach into the realm of possibility. For the plan to be successful, it was mandatory that highly trained personnel be in constant attendance. Once a lethal arrhythmia was detected by the observer, the rhythm disturbance could be terminated instantly and death prevented. Furthermore, these trained personnel would also be able to detect the earliest signs of other complications (particularly circulatory failure) and start treatment for these complications promptly. In this way, the number of deaths from these other causes could also be reduced.

These principles formed the basis of the original concept of intensive coronary care.

22

THE SYSTEM OF INTENSIVE CORONARY CARE

Intensive coronary care is a *system* for preventing death from the complications of acute myocardial infarction, primarily by means of *specialized nursing care*. The concept is based on a *physician-nurse team* approach to care.

The total system of care is shown in the following diagram.

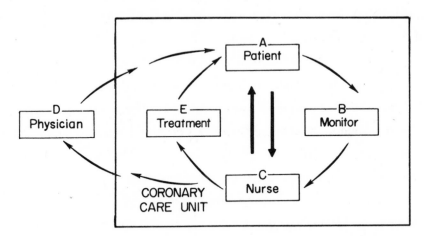

The patient (A) with a suspected acute myocardial infarction is admitted directly to the coronary care unit where all equipment and material necessary for the detection and treatment of the complications of acute myocardial infarction are centralized. The unit is self-sufficient.

Monitoring equipment (B), attached to the patient, displays continuous electrocardiographic information on an oscilloscope. In this way, the rhythm of the heart (and the development of arrhythmias) is apparent at all times. The cardiac monitors also include rate meters which indicate the minute-to-minute heart rate and alarm systems which alert personnel to changes in the heart rate. If the rate of the heart exceeds, or falls below pre-set levels, an alarm is triggered.

The nurse (C), who has been specifically trained for this specialized role, is in constant attendance within the unit. She is able to interpret the electrocardiographic information displayed on the oscilloscope and is aware of the significance of changes in rate and rhythm. In addition, the nurse must repeatedly assess the clinical condition of the patient at the bedside by planned, careful observation in order to detect signs of other complications of myocardial infarction. In the event of a change in the patient's status, either clinically or electrocardiographically, the nurse must decide upon a course of action which may involve either further observation, notifying a physician, or immediate direct action on her own (including defibrillation).

The physician (D), unlike the nurse, is not in constant attendance. He relies, fundamentally, on the observations made by the nurse member of the team who advises him of changes in the clinical course. That the physician delegates unusual authority to the nurse in this team approach to care is one of the most distinguishing characteristics of the system of intensive coronary care.

The **treatment program** (E), directed by the physician, is designed to prevent lethal complications. In the original plan of intensive coronary care the focus of the treatment program was on *resuscitation* from death-producing arrhythmias; at the present time, the emphasis is on *prevention* of arrhythmias and other complications. (See page 28).

It is essential to view the concept of intensive coronary care as a *system*. As with any effective system, optimal function is achieved by the interrelationship of its various components; individually, the components have little meaning and cannot produce the desired effect. For this reason, it should be apparent that monitoring equipment alone, regardless of its design or elegance, cannot be construed as intensive coronary care. An impression exists (perhaps because of the human tendency to upgrade the performance of electronic machines) that these devices are self-sufficient and can reliably "watch" the patient's heart and accurately sound alarms when catastrophes occur. On this basis, it has been reasoned by some, that physicians and nurses could work elsewhere in the hospital and yet respond to alarm situations and save patients' lives. This scheme which would obviate the need for continuous nursing care and other elements of the system, has no merit and will be of minimal help at best. Monitoring equipment alone does not warrant its expense.

Constant, specialized, nursing care is absolutely essential in the system and there can be no compromise with this need. *In fact, the nurse is the key to the entire program of coronary care.* The enormity of her role should be appreciated. It is readily apparent that the nurse has multiple responsibilities in this system of care; to fulfill these she requires unique skills most of which were unknown to nursing in the past. Nurses who serve in this specialized setting must have a usable knowledge of electrocardiography with the ability to recognize all significant arrhythmias. In addition, a clear understanding of the symptoms and clinical findings of the various complications of acute myocardial infarction is essential to detect early warnings of their occurrence, and to follow the patient's clinical course. Finally, the nurse has to be versed in the treatment of arrhythmias and other complications and also be competent in the use of all necessary equipment. Most importantly, the nurse will have to perform life-saving techniques (e.g., defibrillation) by herself under certain circumstances.

This advanced concept of nursing care implies much more than simply having a nurse stationed in a coronary unit whose basic responsibility is merely to call a physician if a monitor alarm sounds. For intensive coronary care to be fully effective, the nurse must assess each problem by herself and assume a *decision-making* role. Unless the nurse is delegated appropriate authority to act on her own the system of care is weakened markedly.

SELECTION OF PATIENTS FOR INTENSIVE CORONARY CARE

If possible, *all* patients with suspected acute myocardial infarction should be treated in a coronary care unit. Admittedly, those patients who show evidence of complications on admission have a far greater chance of developing additional problems than those who are free of complications at the time of arrival and it might be argued that this comprehensive, expensive care should be reserved for only those who are acutely ill when first seen. However, this reasoning is fallacious, because the subsequent clinical course of patients with acute myocardial infarction is by no means predictable. *Many patients who appear perfectly stable on admission, may be candidates for sudden death.* This threat is apparent from the following table where the frequency of complications and the death rate among patients with no complications (so-called "good-risk" patients) at the time of admission are shown.

The Clinical Course of 57 "good-risk" Patients

(Patients admitted with no major complications)

Incidence of Complications*

Congestive heart failure		7
Cardiogenic shock		5
Major arrhythmias		30
Ventricular fibrillation or cardiac standstill (ventricular asystole)	5	
Other major arrhythmias	25	
Embolic phenomena		0
Ruptured ventricle		0
Deaths		5 (8.8%)

*Some patients had more than one complication.

Based on evidence of this type it is quite clear that *any* patient with acute myocardial infarction, regardless of his clinical status at the time of admission, should be treated in a coronary care unit.

Many patients are admitted to hospitals because of chest pain, or other symptoms, creating suspicion of acute myocardial infarction, but a positive diagnosis of this disease cannot be established at the time because the electrocardiogram fails to show the typical changes of acute infarction. A decision must be made about whether these patients with *suspected* (but not proven) infarction should be admitted to the coronary care unit or observed elsewhere in the hospital until a definitive diagnosis is established. Experience has shown that patients with suspected attacks should be treated within the coronary care unit as if infarction had actually occurred. If this practice is followed, in approximately 25 to 30% of all patients admitted to the unit, the diagnosis of acute myocardial infarction will not be confirmed because either another diagnosis (e.g., acute cholecystitis) becomes apparent, or because the problem was coronary insufficiency rather than true infarction. While this plan may superficially appear wasteful in terms of space, personnel, and equipment, it is nevertheless a sound principle because of the bewildering speed in which lethal complications may develop among these patients. Any compromise with this approach is a flirtation with danger.

THE DURATION OF INTENSIVE CORONARY CARE

The average duration of stay in most coronary care units is 5 days. This period of time has been chosen because of evidence (Fig. 1) which showed that the major incidence of death among patients hospitalized with acute myocardial infarction occurs within this period.

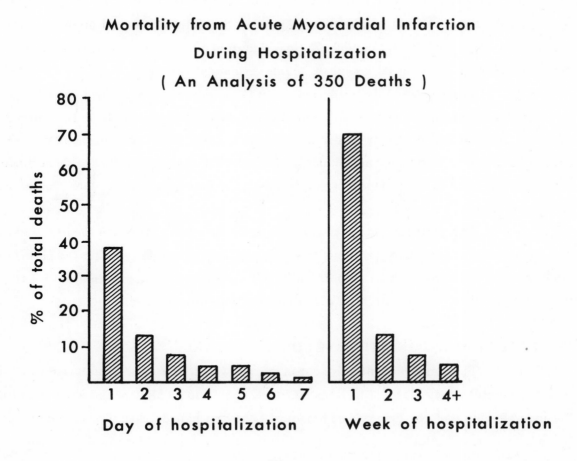

Fig. 1

It is apparent that approximately 40% of all deaths take place within the initial 24 hours after admission, and 62% of the mortality occurs within the first 3 days. After this critical period of 72 hours, the fatality decreases sharply; by the end of the first week of hospitalization more that 70% of all deaths have occurred. After this time the death rate averages 1-2% per day, a yield that may not be commensurate with the effort and expense involved in this highly specialized care during these latter days. Many hospitals prefer to limit the stay in the coronary care unit to only 3 days with the realization that the majority of deaths will have occurred by then. By shortening the intensive care period, more patients can be accommodated within the facility. Five days of intensive coronary care seems to be a sensible compromise.

It can be argued that since complications are not predictable and may occur at any time after the infarction that patients should receive this intensive care throughout the entire hospital period. This is not a feasible approach for several reasons. First, the unit would have to be inordinately large to accommodate all patients with myocardial infarction for this length of time. (Surveys have shown that approximately 8% of a total hospital census on any given day are patients with acute myocardial infarction; in a 300 bed institution the facility would require about 25 beds.) Secondly, prolonged intensive care is prohibitively expensive to the patient. A final deterrent to extended intensive care is the adverse psychological effects it may create among certain patients.

Recognizing these problems, many hospitals have established *intermediate care* (or sub-acute) facilities to combat the problem of death after transfer from the coronary care unit. While it is true that most deaths from acute myocardial occur in the first several days, the mortality during the remainder of the hospital stay is nevertheless disturbingly high, and it is clear that a program of graduated care is necessary if these "late" deaths are to be prevented.

The plan for subacute care generally involves a separate facility usually contiguous with the coronary care unit to which patients are transferred after the period of intensive care. The subacute unit permits additional surveillance of these patients in a setting that is intermediate between intensive care and customary hospital care.

THE EFFECTIVENESS OF INTENSIVE CORONARY CARE

The concept of intensive coronary care was first proposed and tested in 1962 by Day at the Bethany Hospital in Kansas City, Kansas, and by Meltzer and Kitchell at the Presbyterian-University of Pennsylvania Medical Center in Philadelphia. The system of care immediately proved effective and the mortality rates were lowered significantly in the two institutions. Both teams of investigators reported that the mortality was reduced by approximately 35% as a result of this specialized care. Specifically, the existing hospital death rates fell from about 30-35% to 20%. The plan of care was immediately accepted throughout the world and hundreds, and then thousands, of coronary care units were soon established. The effectiveness of the system of care was promptly confirmed and a similar reduction in mortality was apparent in most institutions. Typical results achieved with the original system of coronary care are as follows:

Series	Place	Number of Patients	Hospital Mortality
Day & Averill	Kansas City	280	20.0%
Meltzer & Kitchell	Philadelphia	500	18.0%
Lown et al.	Boston	300	17.7%
Julian & Oliver	Scotland	552	19.2%
Killip & Kimball	New York	300+	21.0%
Sloman et al.	Australia	350	18.0%

To assess the effectiveness of intensive coronary care more specifically, a study was conducted at the Presbyterian-University of Pennsylvania Medical Center in which patients with suspected myocardial infarction were assigned *randomly* to either the coronary unit or to customary hospital rooms. If a vacancy existed in the 3-bed coronary care unit when the patient reached the hospital, he was admitted directly to this facility and designated as a *study* patient. If the beds were occupied at the time, the patient was assigned to regular hospital quarters and categorized as a *control* subject.

Patients admitted to the CCU were treated by a well-organized team of physicians and nurses. The control cases received the customary good care offered in a university-affiliated hospital. At the end of 96 hours, patients in the coronary care unit were transferred to usual hospital facilities and received standard care. Those patients originally admitted to customary rooms remained there throughout their hospital stay.·

During a 20-month period, 441 patients with suspected acute myocardial infarction were admitted to the hospital. After excluding 27% of these patients because the diagnosis of acute myocardial infarction could not be confirmed, there were 181 patients in the study group and 131 in the control category. Statistical analysis revealed that the study and control patients were similar in all respects (age, sex, type of infarction, etc.) - as would be expected with a random distribution - and therefore a valid comparison could be made between the two groups of patients.

The respective mortality rates were as follows:

Number of Patients	Mortality at 96 hours	Mortality at Discharge
Study (181)	12.0%	19.9%
Control (131)	20.8%	30.8%

From this research study it was apparent that *patients treated during the first four days in a coronary care unit had a mortality about 33% less than those receiving usual hospital care.*

The basis of the decrease in the death rate resulting from intensive coronary care was readily apparent: the system was capable of preventing nearly all sudden deaths from *arrhythmias.* However, it was not effective in saving lives from the other complications of acute myocardial infarction. In particular, the mortality from cardiogenic shock and acute cardiac failure showed no significant improvement compared to the expected rate without intensive coronary care. It was clear that if any further reduction in the death rate was to be achieved, a different approach would be needed to combat circulatory failure.

THE CURRENT CONCEPT OF INTENSIVE CORONARY CARE

During the past few years, the original system of intensive coronary care has undergone at least two important changes:

1) It became apparent that the death producing arrhythmias, ventricular fibrillation and ventricular standstill, seldom occurred spontaneously; instead, these catastrophic events were almost always preceded by lesser, *warning* arrhythmias. *By recognizing and treating warning arrhythmias it was found that lethal arrhythmias could be prevented.* The emphasis of the system of coronary care then changed from resuscitation to prevention of death-producing arrhythmias. It is now clear that if lesser arrhythmias are controlled by vigorous treatment, primary ventricular fibrillation and ventricular standstill can be averted in most instances. This concept has become the cornerstone of current-day coronary care.

2) Because of the inability of the original system of coronary care to control deaths due to cardiogenic shock and circulatory failure, it became evident that a different attack was needed against these complications. Perhaps the most meaningful step in this direction to date involves more *aggressive management* of the failing heart. The program includes deliberate detection of the earliest signs of heart failure (by careful observation and appropriate clinical studies) followed by specific, planned therapy. The aim of this plan is to attempt to limit the extent of circulatory failure and hopefully to prevent its progression before irreversible changes occur.

CHAPTER 4

The Coronary Care Unit

GENERAL CONSIDERATIONS

Although the concept of intensive coronary care has already been proven remarkably effective in practice and it now appears that most hospitals will ultimately have these specialized facilities, there are nevertheless certain possible deterrents that should be recognized before a hospital attempts to implement the full system of coronary care.

The following questions should be answered:

1) Are nurses available to staff the unit?

   As explained in the next chapter, nurses who serve in coronary care units must have distinct qualifications and training. Unless an adequate number of nurses of this caliber are available, or can be recruited, the program of intensive coronary care (as described here) should not be undertaken and a modified plan of care must be adopted. *Ascertaining the availability of nurses is absolutely essential and should precede any other planning.*

   Only those hospitals which have a trained staff of nurses can rightfully claim to offer intensive coronary care; other institutions, simply have coronary care units. There is a major difference between these two concepts.

2) Are there enough patients with acute myocardial infarction admitted each year to justify establishing a system of intensive care?

   Unless there are at least 100 admissions yearly (an average of 2 per week) with myocardial infarction, the expense, allocation of space and the diversion of personnel may not be warranted. In these circumstances, the system of care may have to be modified.

3) Are the medical and nursing staffs and the administration willing to accept the fact that the coronary care unit must be autonomous to be successful?

   For the system of intensive coronary care to function optimally it is essential that the beds within the unit be used solely for patients with proven or suspected myocardial infarction. In these days of hospital overcrowding there is often temptation to fill those beds designated for coronary care with other patients not having acute infarction in order to meet demands. Because the system of coronary care is predicated on readiness and preparedness, this latter alternative of occupying empty beds because of their availability is completely destructive to the program and its results.

4) Can the hospital and its clientele afford this type of care?

Admittedly, economic considerations are a tragic reason for denying a hospital or a community this specialized care but the expense of coronary care is very high and this fact must be realistically considered. Present estimates suggest that the average cost per day per patient in a CCU is the equivalent of 3 private duty nurses daily in addition to the normal per diem cost of a hospital room. The major item of this expense (which may amount to as much as $100-$150 a day or more in some hospitals) is personnel.

Assuming these basic problems are surmountable, consideration should then be given to the size of the unit, its design and equipment, and its staff.

SIZE OF THE UNIT

Bed Capacity. While the actual number of beds for a unit depends on the demands of the community (as well as financial considerations), as a general rule a five bed unit will be the most efficient and economical size for a hospital with 200 admissions per year for acute myocardial infarction, with an average stay in the unit of five days. Obviously if there are more admissions per year, or if the period of intensive care will be longer, the bed capacity of the unit must be increased proportionately.

In planning the actual bed capacity for the unit it is wise to review the specific number of patients admitted to the hospital with acute myocardial infarction during the preceding two or three years. This figure is a much better index of the anticipated needs of a hospital than its total bed capacity or total annual admission rate. (Community hospitals, serving large suburban or rural geographic areas often have a relatively higher percentage of admissions with acute myocardial infarctions than larger urban hospitals and may actually require porportionately more coronary care beds on this basis).

A general formula for calculating the number of beds required for a unit is as follows:

1) Determine the number of patients discharged from the hospital in the previous year with the diagnosis of acute myocardial infarction.

2) Multiply this number by the average stay anticipated in the unit (5 days is the average figure in most institutions).

3) Divide this product by 365, giving the daily bed requirement for patients with proven infarction.

4) Multiply this quotient by 2. This latter step is essential because in a high percentage of patients admitted to the unit, the admission diagnosis of myocardial infarction will not be confirmed (these admissions would not be evident from statistics of discharge diagnoses).

For example, if in the previous year, 200 patients were discharged with the diagnosis of acute myocardial infarction, the bed capacity for the proposed unit could be calculated in the following manner:

$$\frac{200 \times 5}{365} = 2.7 \times 2 = 5.4 \text{ beds}$$

Thus, a 5 or 6 bed unit should be planned for this institution.

Dimensions of the Unit. While the ultimate size of the unit is most often determined by the space that can be made available within the hospital, an ideal unit of 5 beds should contain a total of at least 1,200 - 1,500 square feet of floor space. Each room in the unit should have approximately 150 square feet with no dimension being less that 12 feet. In addition to these rooms, adequate space must also be provided for a nursing station; storage and supply: drug cabinets; resuscitative equipment; and other specialized devices.

A representative floor plan of a five bed unit is shown in Fig.2.

PHYSICAL DESIGN OF THE UNIT

Although a detailed description of the physical design of a coronary care unit is beyond the intent of this manual, it is nevertheless relevant that nurses have a general concept of some of the basic problems involved in planning such a facility. This knowledge is useful, particularly when nurses are asked to participate in the designing of new units. The following factors are considered pertinent.

1) Ideally, the unit should be composed of a series of individual private rooms. Open-ward type facilities, with curtains or partitions between beds, are unsuitable for providing the peacefulness and serenity required in the overall treatment program. The goal in design should be to ensure that individual patients remain unaware of each other. It has been shown that when distinct separation of patients does not exist, emergency situations occurring in adjacent areas may have an adverse effect on the surrounding patients.

2) Similarly, the unit should be designed so that beds and litters can be moved to and from the individual rooms without the risk of disturbing

32

Floor Plan of a 5-Bed Coronary Care Unit

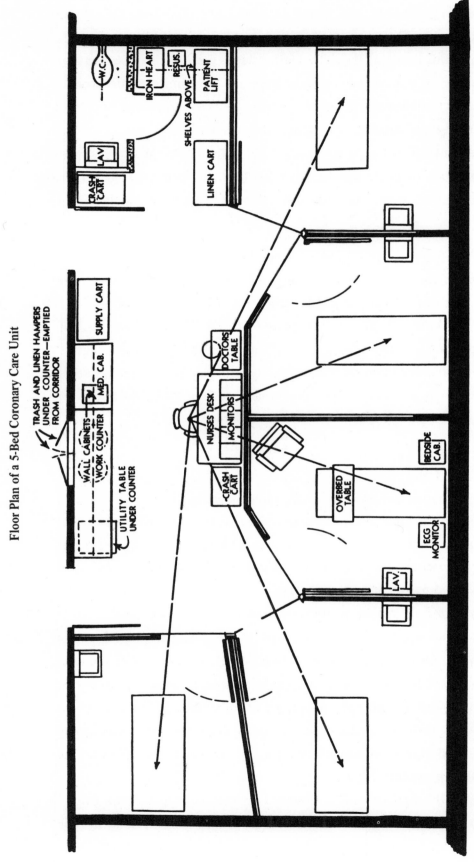

Fig. 2

A CORONARY CARE UNIT: 5-BEDS

U.S. DEPARTMENT OF HEALTH, EDUCATION, AND WELFARE
PUBLIC HEALTH SERVICE
DIVISION OF HOSPITAL AND MEDICAL FACILITIES

PRELIMINARY

SCALE: ¼"=1'-0"

*This diagram is reproduced from *A Facility for Coronary Care* published by the Division of Medical and Hospital Facilities of the United States Public Health Service (PHS publication #1250). This pamphlet offers excellent advice about the physical design of a coronary unit and should be consulted by those seeking detailed planning information. A second valuable directive for planning coronary care units is Guidelines For Coronary Care Units (Public Health publication #1824 July 1968) published by Heart Disease and Stroke Control Program of the U. S. Public Health Service. Both pamphlets are for sale by the Superintendent of Documents, U. S. Government Printing Office, Washington, D. C., 20402.

the other patients in the unit. This unobtrusive movement is particularly important when deaths occur.

3) All beds should be directly visible from the central nursing station if at all feasible. Direct visual observation is an integral part of coronary care nursing and it is most undesirable to rely on monitor surveillance as the prime means of patient assessment. Some hospitals have utilized closed television circuits from patient rooms to the nursing station as a method of overseeing patients when space limitation prevents direct vision. This technique is less-than-desirable and is usually an unfortunate compromise from the patient's standpoint. In very large units more than one nursing station may be required to provide direct observation of all patients.

4) Patients' rooms should be at least 12 x 12 feet in size to allow adequate space for equipment and for multiple personnel (particularly at the time of emergencies). Since many of the patients in the unit will not be desperately ill and will be there primarily for observation, it is necessary that the unit be attractively and cheerfully decorated with this fact in mind. A window should be present in each room; "inside" rooms are very depressing to patients. Provisions for noise control should be recognized and acoustical materials for ceilings and floors should be used whenever possible. It is wise to furnish each room with clocks, calendars, radio and music so that the patient does not become separated from his normal environment.

5) It is beneficial to locate the coronary care unit at a site contiguous with, or nearby, the hospital's general intensive care facility. This arrangement allows for sharing of certain basic facilities and services (utility rooms, pantries, storage areas, etc.) that would otherwise require duplication.

On the other hand, it is not wise to actually combine these two types of units into one facility served by a single staff. (There is good reason to believe that the nursing staff of a coronary care unit must be full-time within the unit and should not be diverted to other areas). Furthermore, the general intensive care unit is usually much too hectic a setting for patients with acute myocardial infarction.

A more important consideration in choosing the location of the CCU is to have the unit as close as possible to the emergency or receiving ward of the hospital. Tragically, many deaths occur during transit to the coronary unit. This threat can be reduced by minimizing the distance between the admission area and the unit.

6) In the design plan it is worthwhile to provide certain additional rooms for purposes other that patient care. Of especial importance are the following areas:

A waiting room for families. Because of the abrupt and critical nature of this illness it is understandable that families will gather and remain near the patient for prolonged periods. Unless provisions are made to accommodate these visitors in a separate room outside the unit, there tends to be much disturbance and congestion at the nurses' station and patient care areas. The family room should have adequate telephone facilities.

A nurses' lounge. Since nursing personnel must be in continuous attendance within the unit it is important that a room be allocated within the unit for the nursing staff. This lounge should include bathroom facilities, lockers, and comfortable furniture.

A physicians' consultation room. While certainly less essential than the two areas just described, a separate room for the use of physicians has proved very useful in many institutions. This space provides not only an office for physicians but also can serve as sleeping quarters when necessary.

7) Air conditioning and an efficient ventilatory system are mandatory, not only for patient and nurse comfort, but also for the proper upkeep of the monitoring equipment. Many of the monitoring systems and other equipment are heat-sensitive and proper room temperature must be maintained to ensure satisfactory function.

8) Multiple, separately fused, electrical outlets are absolutely essential and should be considered in the early stages of planning. Approximately eight, *grounded* outlets are required for each bed.

Electrical grounding within the unit must have unquestionable integrity. Unless true and effective grounding is provided, a potential danger of patient electrocution exists, particularly when several electrical devices are used simultaneously. Grounding which involves no more than connecting a wire to a convenient water or heating pipe is wholly inadequate, nor is a "three-pronged" plug, by itself, a real safety measure. *A true common grounding circuit is totally essential.*

Because of the increasing use of major electrical equipment within units (including portable x-ray machines) 220 volt lines should be incorporated in the electrical planning. An emergency power supply should be available in the event of electrical failure of the primary circuit.

9) Effective communication and alarm systems are required for all units. These systems should permit the nursing staff to summon help promptly and directly. The usual hospital communication network, which involves the circuitous chain of dialing the operator, paging of physicians and returning the call to the unit, results in too much delay. A special alarm signal, or code, initiated directly by the nurse in the unit which bypasses the customary route is very desirable.

EQUIPMENT FOR THE CORONARY CARE UNIT

For General care

1) Electrical beds with proper grounding
2) Bedside commodes (or "Pullman" toilets).
3) Blood pressure apparatus, wall mounted, at each bedside.
4) Metal rods, suspended from the ceiling to hang intravenous solutions, instead of the familiar floor standards.
5) An effective lighting system for each bed including a separate small "spotlight."

For Cardiac Monitoring

One cardiac monitor, consisting of an oscilloscope, rate meter, and alarm mechanism, is required for each patient. (The specific details of monitoring devices are considered in Chapter 6.)

The decision about the type and the location of the electrocardiographic monitoring system depends basically on the size of the unit and its design. Among the alternatives are the following: a) to have the electrocardiographic monitors centralized in the nurses station with no detection equipment in the patient's room; b) to have individual monitors at each bedside with "slave" oscilloscopes and alarm systems in the central nursing area; or c) to have the individual monitors at the nurses' station with the "slave" attachments at the bedsides. The last plan is probably the most valuable; it combines the advantage of the patient not being aware of the business of monitoring with its inherent problems (false alarms, lead failures, etc.) and at the same time allows those attending the patient to observe the electrocardiogram at the bedside without returning to the central station. This latter aspect is important during emergency situations (e.g., defibrillation) and avoids the necessity of leaving the patient to ascertain the effectiveness of treatment.

For Clinical Assesment

1) A portable x-ray machine is extremely useful for detecting early heart failure and should be readily available for use in the coronary care unit.

2) Hemodynamic measurements are employed frequently in the CCU and apparatus for these purposes should be on hand. This includes manometers and appropriate plastic tubing for determination of central venous pressure and intra-arterial pressure.

3) The unit requires a separate electrocardiographic machine for taking 12 lead tracings for diagnostic purposes. The machine is also used to document various arrhythmias seen on the oscilloscope if the monitoring equipment itself does not have a direct ECG write-out device.

For Treatment and Resuscitation

1) A defibrillator should be present at all times at *each* bedside. While this number of defibrillators may seem redundant, the safety and assurance afforded by these individual devices certainly justifies their cost. Lesser numbers are not without risk.

2) At least three pacemakers (battery-operated, demand type) along with appropriate pacing catheters for transvenous (and transthoracic) use are required for each five-bed unit.

3) Respiratory assistance equipment should be permanently available in the unit. Manual breathing bags and a mechanical respirator, preferably a pressure cycled machine, are essential.

4) A "crash cart" which contains all supplies, equipment, and drugs needed for emergencies and resuscitative attempts. This cart should be easily moveable and be constructed of heavy gauge stainless steel with a low center of gravity to prevent tipping. Preferably the cart should contain 3 or more shelves, the topmost of which can serve as a work area.
   Separate drawers for drug storage are located between the first and second shelves. The equipment and supplies customarily contained in a "crash cart" are listed in Table 1 at the end of the chapter.

5) A dependable oxygen supply, preferably "piped in" from a central source is mandatory. Face masks and nasal cannulas should be present at each bedside for immediate use.

6) An effective system for aspiration and suction should be available along

with a laryngoscope and various endotracheal tubes.

7) A bed board (or cafeteria tray) should be located at each bedside for use during closed chest cardiac massage.

8) An automatic timing device - set for a two minute period - which the nurse activates at the onset of cardiac arrest, is useful.

9) Tourniquets, in the form of either plain rubber tubing or an automatic rotating tourniquet machine, are required for treatment of acute pulmonary edema.

10) Prepared trays (packages) for venous cut-down, urinary catheterization and tracheostomy should be stored in the unit.

DRUGS REQUIRED IN THE CORONARY CARE UNIT

A specific drug list for the unit should be established and adequate amounts of these medications should be on hand at all times. One nurse should be responsible for their inventory, availability and re-order.

It is essential that these drugs be stored in an orderly way so that they can be located instantly without the need for searching for a particular drug at the most inopportune time. The choice of drugs for the unit will vary to some extent with the preferences of the physicians at individual hospitals. The drug list employed at the Presbyterian-University of Pennsylvania Medical Center is listed in Table 2.

TABLE 1

EQUIPMENT AND SUPPLIES FOR CRASH CART

Top Shelf

defibrillator
electrode paste
syringes (5cc, 10cc, 50cc)
needles (#18, 20, 21, & 25)
intracardiac needles (#22)
intravenous catheters (angio-cath)
scalp-vein set
intravenous tubing and adapters
    (venopak, minidrip, etc.)
tourniquets for venipuncture
alcohol sponges
airway and padded tongue blades
adhesive tape
a tray containing:
    lidocaine 2%
    isoproterenol 1cc vials
    water for injection
    saline for injection

Shelf 2

ambu bag and tubing
sterile gloves and drapes
endotracheal tray (tube, adaptors, airway,
    and laryngoscope)
pacemaker
pacemaker catheters (transvenous and transthoracic)
cut down tray
suction catheters
central venous pressure set

Shelf 3

500 ml 5% dextrose in water
500 ml 5% sodium bicarbonate solution
1000 ml 5% dextrose in water
solution administration sets
arm board
tracheotomy set
sterile (4 x 4) dressings
rotating tourniquets

In drawers

sodium bicarbonate	50cc	5 amps
digoxin	0.5mg	6 amps
cedilanid	0.8mg	2 amps
ouabain	0.5mg	4 amps
Levophed	4cc	2 amps
Aramine	100mg	3 amps
Wyamine	30mg	3 amps
Isuprel	1mg	4 amps
aminophylline	500mg	3 amps
Pronestyl	10cc	3 amps
sodium amytal	500mg	1 amp
Brevital	500mg	1 vial
Valium	10mg	2 amps
atropine sulfate	0.4mg	1 vial
Lasix	20mg	1 amp
Edecrin	50mg	1 amp
Solu-Cortef	100mg	2 amps
calcium gluconate	10ml	1 amp
Inderal	1mg/cc	1 amp
mannitol	12.5gm	1 amp

TABLE 2

DRUGS STOCKED IN THE CORONARY CARE UNIT

AT THE PRESBYTERIAN-UNIVERSITY OF PENNSYLVANIA MEDICAL CENTER

Anti-Arrhythmic Agents
Lidocaine
Procaineamide (Pronestyl)
Quinidine
Atropine
Isoproterenol (Isuprel)
Disodium EDTA (Endrate Sodium)
Propanolol HCL (Inderal)
Diphenylhydantoin (Dilantin)
Potassium chloride
Prostigmin (neostigmine)

Anti-Coagulants
Heparin
Warfarin sodium
Dicumarol

Anti-Coagulant Antagonists
Vitamin K_1 oxide (Mephyton)
Protamine sulfate

Anti-Emetics
Trimethobenzamine HCL (Tigan)
Perchlorperazine (Compazine)
Dramamine

Anti-Hypertensives
Reserpine

Bronchodilators
Aminophylline

Coronary Dilators
Nitroglycerin

Digitalis Preparations
Digoxin
Ouabain
Cedilanid

Diuretic Agents
Furosemide (Lasix)
Ethacrynic acid (Edecrin)
Sodium mercaptomerin (Thiomerin)
Thiazides
Mannitol

Electrolyte Solutions
Sodium bicarbonate
1/6 molar lactate
Calcium gluconate
Potassium chloride

Intra Venous Solutions
5% glucose in water
10% glucose in water
5% glucose in PSS

Narcotics
Meperidine HCL (Demerol)
Morphine SO4
Hydromorphone (Dilaudid)

Narcotic Antagonist
Nalline

Plasma Expanders
Dextran solution

Sedatives
Sodium amytal
Sodium methohexitol (Brevital)
Phenobarbital

Steroids and Hormones
Prednisone
Hydrocortisone
Insulin

Tranquilizers
Diazepon (Valium)
Chlordiazepoxide HCL (Librium)
Promazine parnoate (Vistaril)
Meprobamate

Vaso-Dilators
Phentolamine (Regitine)
Chlorpromazine (Thorazine)
Phenoxybenzamine HCL (Dibenzyline)

Vasopressor Agents
Epinephrine
Nor-epinephrine (Levophed)
Metariminol bitartrate (Aramine)
Mephentermine SO_4 (Wyamine)
Methoxamine (Vasoxyl)
Phenylephrine HCL (Neo-Synephrine)

CHAPTER 5

The Staff of the Coronary Care Unit and the Nurses' Training Program

It is absolutely essential that the care of patients in a coronary unit be delegated to a *team* of physicians and nurses. In fact, the team approach is the most distinguishing characteristic of the coronary care concept. Because all of the members of the team understand the aims of care and recognize their respective responsibilities and functions, the effectiveness of the system of care is markedly enhanced. Furthermore, a team effort develops clarity of communication and a mutual respect among the individual members. Unless the physicians and nurses in a coronary care unit function as an *organized team,* the ultimate result of the entire program will prove very disappointing.

The ideal CCU team is composed of a) a director, b) attending physicians, (and, in some hospitals, the intern and resident staff), c) a group of nurses specifically trained in the principles and practices of coronary care nursing.

DIRECTOR OF THE UNIT

As with any successful team effort, one person must be in charge and serve as its responsible member and representative. Ideally, the director should be a cardiologist or an internist who has the knowledge, dedication, interest, and time to coordinate the whole program. The general duties and responsibilities of the director are:

a) to assume authority and responsibility for establishing basic policies of the unit in terms of the admission of patients, length of stay in unit, physicians' privileges, etc.

b) to establish the system of care (including the treatment plan to be employed) in the unit, and to delegate specific duties to the respective members of the team.

c) to supervise and participate in the training program for nurses (and other members) who comprise the CCU team.

d) to choose and be responsible for the equipment and material used in the unit.

e) to serve as liaison between the attending staff, the hospital administration, and the members of the CCU team regarding policies or other problems that arise.

f) to assume command of patient care when critical situations occur in the absence of the attending physician.

g) to evaluate the effectiveness of the unit and the various practices employed periodically.

h) to serve as consultant to the attending physician upon request.

ATTENDING PHYSICIANS

It is generally agreed that the care of the patient in the CCU should be supervised by his own physician. The director of the unit and the other members of the team essentially assist the attending physician in this case but do not displace him or assume his role. However, it is essential that the attending physician be willing to delegate some of his normal responsibility to the other team members. In particular, the attending physician must transfer certain authority to the nurse so that she can assume a decision-making role on her own when the situation demands.

The delegation of authority from one physician to another physician in the coronary care unit has broad implications and the extent of this practice varies considerably at different hospitals. In some institutions, this delegation of authority involves no more than an agreement that any physician who happens to be present at the time of a catastrophe may assume command (e.g., defibrillate a patient of another physician). In other hospitals, the director of the unit, or a committee of physicians are empowered to act in their own right, not only in the event of emergencies, but also if the general treatment program prescribed by the attending physician fails to meet the standards of the unit.

Attending physicians should participate in the ongoing training program for nurses (and house officers). His presence at team conferences is especially important when the patients to be discussed are under his care.

THE INTERN AND RESIDENT STAFF

In many hospitals, interns and resident physicians become part of the coronary care team as delegates of the attending physician. It should be recognized that these house officers are in training and that their primary function is not to replace the attending physician in the direct care of the patients; their assignment to the coronary care unit is meant as an educational experience.

It is a customary practice in many hospitals for a house officer to be notified when the CCU nurse detects a change in the patient's clinical status, or if a life-threatening situation occurs. It is the decision he makes at these times that often means the difference between life and death. In many instances, the house officer will have time to confer with the attending physician or the unit director before deciding on a course of action, but with catastrophic situations, the resident physician alone makes the ultimate decision of treatment; therefore, his role is vitally important to the success of the entire program. Certain aspects regarding house officer training and responsibilities are worth considering.

1) The house officer must receive detailed instruction in the system of coronary care; it is unwise to assume that their existent knowledge of myocardial infarction is sufficient for the demands of this specialized care. The house officers' training should include:

a) a review of arrhythmias using slides or actual ECG tracing.

b) practical experience with the use of monitors, pacemakers, defibrillators and equipment for assisted respiration.

c) the recognition of, and treatment program for, complications of acute myocardial infarction.

d) the pharmacology of anti-arrhythmic and other cardiac drugs.

e) the use of various techniques for hemodynamic measurements.

f) methods of cardiopulmonary resuscitation.

2) The unique role of the CCU nurse and her status on the team should be carefully explained to the house staff. As might be anticipated, the traditional physician-nurse relationship may become distorted in this setting where the nurse is assuming duties and responsibilities beyond those generally expected of nurses. Not infrequently, because of their constant exposure to the problems related to myocardial infarction, these nurses become remarkably competent in this area and the wise house officer will recognize their judgement and experience.

3) An on-call schedule for the house staff should be established and posted daily, in a conspicuous site, so that the nurse knows which physician to call for advice or for emergencies during each shift. Preferably two physicians should be listed for both day and night tours. This type of call system is more effective than having the nurse sound a general alarm which can be answered by any physician who happens to be nearby. This latter alternative tends to create confusion with the sudden assemblage of several members of the house staff, but without one person to make decisions.

4) House officers and the nursing staff should *jointly* make daily rounds on the patients in the unit. In this way, patient problems, not apparent to

individual members of the team, can be identified and solved together. This form of communication is of great importance if effective care is to result.

THE NURSE MEMBERS OF THE TEAM

Size and Composition of the Nursing Staff

For optimum effectiveness, a coronary care unit should have a ratio of one professional nurse for every two or three patients. Therefore, a 4 to 6 bed unit would require two nurses per shift and a total nursing staff of at least 10 to 12 nurses (including relief shifts). Because this high nurse-patient ratio may be unrealistic in many hospitals, the number of professional nurses can be reduced by the use of licensed practical nurses who can take care of feeding, bed changing, bathing, and other lesser tasks for several patients, under the supervision of the staff nurse. While this latter alternative is commonly employed by necessity, the fact remains that the presence of the professional nurse at the bedside is invaluable in terms of assessing the patient's clinical status by repeated, thoughtful observation and for the security she is able to impart to the patient. Whenever possible, professional nurses should staff the unit. This does not imply that highly motivated, specially trained, licensed practical nurses cannot be of great value in relieving the professional nurse of some bedside nursing care; in fact, it is appropriate to include them in portions of the training program offered for professional nurses.

Selection of Nurses for the Unit

Despite the current nursing shortage and the problem of staffing hospitals, let alone specialized units, it is nevertheless essential that the CCU nurses be deliberately chosen rather than merely accepted because of their availability or willingness; under no circumstances should nurses be forced or coerced to work in a coronary care unit. In view of the time and effort involved in their training and the extraordinary responsibilities which they assume, it is particularly important that certain basic requirements be met by prospective candidates. The criteria that we have found most reliable in selecting CCU nurses are as follows:

a) intelligence.

It is quite clear that a high ability to learn, assimilate, and use new material is a prime requisite for nurses chosen to work in the coronary care unit. Recognizing that nurses will require specialized training in unfamiliar subjects, such as electrocardiography, electronic monitoring, precise clinical observation, etc., it is understandable that those nurses who have ranked high in their basic nursing programs are likely to be the best candidates for this exacting role. The selection of nurses with lesser academic backgounds (regardless of their other proficiencies) is probably unwise.

b) **previous nursing experience with acutely ill patients.**

Experience in recovery rooms, general intensive care units, or in the field of heart surgery is extremely vauable preparation and the transition from these areas to coronary care nursing can be made easily by nurses with this background. High intelligence, however, is a more important qualification than such experience.

c) **emotional stability.**

It must be recognized that patients admitted to a coronary care unit are seriously ill and that the death rate among them is much higher than in ordinary hospital facilities. This creates a potentially depressing atmosphere and the prospective nurse should evaluate her personal reaction to this setting and make certain that it will not adversely affect her. Nurses working in a coronary care unit must be able to face the stress of repeated sudden emergencies which are inherent in the very nature of the disease. We have found some nurses, totally competent in other areas of nursing, who were awed by the responsibility of making instant decisions and acting on their own in repeated critical situations. On the positive side, the gratification of the CCU nurses who have saved lives by their own ability is probably unique in their profession.

d) **social maturity.**

As might be expected, coronary care unit nurses soon become distinguished from other nurses in the hospital because of their unusual status and responsibility, as well as their specialized skills and knowledge. Since this may tend to create dissention in the nursing ranks, social maturity is a valuable asset in avoiding this problem. A second source of social concern is the unusual co-professional relationship that exists when nurses and physicians work together as members of a team, particularly when the nurse, rather than the physician, is the key member of the group. It is not uncommon for CCU nurses to become so adept at interpreting arrhythmias and assessing critical situations, that their know-how and judgement often challenge the physician members of the team. It takes considerable discretion and a mature approach for the nurse not to take advantage of this situation.

e) **dedication to bedside nursing.**

Unlike many types of hospital nursing today where the nurse is based at a nursing station and is concerned fundamentally with administrative details, coronary care nursing is wholly involved with direct bedside care. It is, therefore, essential that the nurse enjoy bedside nursing and the inter-personal relationships inherent in this role, rather than fulfilling her responsibilities simply from a sense of duty.

f) **age and health.**

Nurses who have graduated from basic nursing programs within the previous few years are the most adaptable for this role and make the best adjustment to the demands of the exacting work in a coronary care unit. Good health is a vital requisite, since the absence of a CCU nurse because of illness, creates an obvious problem in terms of the limited number of trained colleagues who can replace her.

The Status of the Coronary Care Nurse

By virtue of education, selection, training, unique ability, and the extraordinary responsibility assumed, coronary care nurses have achieved rather high status and prestige among their professional colleagues. While this position is well deserved, there has been an unfortunate tendency in some circles for nurses enjoying this status to isolate themselves from other nurses within the hospital. This separation is disadvantageous for all concerned and should be avoided.

METHODS OF TRAINING CCU NURSES

A nurse cannot function in a coronary care unit solely on the basis of customary undergraduate education. Additional specialized training is essential for this role.

While there are many methods of preparing the nurse for her duties and responsibilities in the coronary care unit, the overall educational program for this purpose can be considered in two phases: the *basic* orientation program and the *on-going* program.

THE BASIC TRAINING PROGRAM

The customary training program for coronary care nursing involves didactic (classroom) instruction, as well as planned clinical (bedside) experience. Basic training is given as an intensive course, usually of four weeks duration, either within an individual hospital or at a regional medical center.

The didactic curriculum generally includes the following subjects:

a) Coronary heart disease

The problem; etiology; epidemiology; risk factors; detection, and natural history.

b) Pathophysiology of acute myocardial infarction

History of attack; physical findings; diagnosis; laboratory studies; pathology; and complications.

c) The cardiovascular system

Anatomy; hemodynamics; electrophysiology; and pharmacology.

d) The coronary care concept

Rationale; the prevention of complications; and the physician-nurse team approach to care.

e) The coronary care unit

Principles and practices; organization and function.

f) Technology

Use of monitoring devices; identification and interpretation of arrhythmias; cardiac pacing; and cardiopulmonary resuscitation.

g) Cardiac nursing

The concept of comprehensive care to meet changing needs; methods of clinical assessment; decision making; patient instruction; and rehabilitation.

In conjuction with classroom instruction, well planned clinical experience is of fundamental importance in the basic training program and must be integrated with the didactic phase of education.

Methods of Basic Training

At the present time, many hospitals are capable of providing effective basic training for their nurses. This implies that the hospital has a functioning coronary care unit and a staff of nurses and physicians who are able and willing to conduct the program. Other institutions are less fortunate in this respect and are unable to offer orientation programs on their own. In these latter circumstances nurses must be sent to established training centers for instruction.

It would serve little purpose here to discuss the diverse training methods employed at large regional centers but it is appropriate to outline some aspects of a *hospital based* orientation program.

A Hospital-Based Orientation Program

Preparation

1) Identify the objectives of the course in terms of the needs of the individual hospital.

2) Select and enlist personnel to teach the course. Of prime importance is the appointment of a capable nurse to serve as director of the teaching program. This teacher should have completed a formal course in coronary care nursing and have had actual clinical experience in an established coronary care unit. Physicians, knowledgeable in the practices of intensive coronary care must also participate in this instructional program.

3) Decide upon, and obtain, various educational materials to be used in presenting the course content. To be considered are: films, slides, arrhythmia teaching equipment, anatomical models, and other teaching aids.

4) Establish a curriculum and a schedule for presentation. The training course should be concentrated over a period of 3-4 weeks. A suggested outline of subject matter is as follows:

An Outline of Didactic Material (A Lecture Series)

1) Orientation to the course.
2) Coronary heart disease: the problem.
3) The concept of intensive coronary care.
4) Anatomy and physiology of the cardiovascular system.
5) Acute myocardial infarction: pathophysiology; diagnosis; and principles of treatment.
6) Nursing care of the patient in a coronary care unit.
7) Psychological aspects of patient care.
8) Principles of cardiac monitoring.
9) Basic electrocardiography.
10) Classification of arrhythmias.
11) Identificaion and interpretation of arrhythmias.
12) Drug treatment of arrhythmias.
13) Electrical treatment of arrhythmias: pacing and cardioversion.
14) The treatment of ventricular fibrillation and ventricular standstill.
15) Cardiopulmonary resuscitation.
16) Assisted respiration and oxygen therapy.
17) Left ventricular failure: diagnosis and treatment.
18) Cardiogenic shock: hemodynamic measurements; diagnosis and treatment.

19) Other complications of acute myocardial infarction; embolism; ventricular rupture; pericarditis; etc.

20) Fluid and electrolyte imbalance.

21) The hospital course after transfer from the unit.

22) Rehabilitation of the patient with myocardial infarction.

23) Course review and final examination.

Methods of Presentation of Didactic Material

The most common plan for presenting the subject matter just described involves an organized lecture series given by members of the medical and nursing staffs of the institution. In conjunction with the lectures, several excellent teaching aids are available to complement the instructional program. These include books of programmed instruction, films, slides, audiotapes, and teaching equipment designed to simulate arrhythmias. More recently, a total, all-inclusive, multimedia instructional system for the training of coronary care nurses has been developed.*

Clinical and Practical Experience

Clinical training in the practices of coronary care is usually obtained at a nurse-to-nurse level with an experienced nurse serving as preceptor. The plan involves much more than simply having the trainee observe her teacher. It should be based on an orderly, planned series of clinical experiences designed to prepare the nurse for her ultimate role. A formal outline for each day should be developed so that the clinical training can be correlated with the didactic material; however, flexibility should be provided by adjusting each day's plan to current circumstances in the unit. For instance, if on the third day of the training program a patient develops a major arrhythmia, it is logical to provide instruction concerning the particular arrhythmia at time of its occurrence rather than at a scheduled, later time. Normally, the clinical program covers a 3-4 week period. Initially, the trainee works with the head nurse (who is usually the preceptor) for two weeks. Following this experience, the trainee is assigned to work with other nurses during the 3 to 11 P.M. tour. If the group of trainees is large, a rotation plan must be established so that overcrowding of the unit is avoided and individual needs are met.

In addition to this form of clinical training, other practical experience can be obtained outside of the coronary care unit. Methods which may be utilized to enable the nurse to become skillful in procedures employed in coronary care nursing include the following:

---

* This training system, which includes motion pictures, sound film strips, audiotapes, texts, problem-solving exercises, as well as outlines of lectures; demonstrations, etc., is based on a research project conducted at the Presbyterian-University of Pennsylvania Medical Center (Grant NU 0096 NIH Division of Nursing) and is commercially available through ROCOM, Nutley, New Jersey.

a) **Electrocardiographic techniques.** Because the mechanics of taking a 12-lead electrocardiogram are difficult to perceive solely from printed material, it is valuable for nurses to accompany the technicians who normally record electrocardiograms throughout the hospital. By performing this procedure among a large group of patients, the nurse soon becomes adept at electrocardiographic techniques.

b) **Laboratory procedures.** Many nurses are not experienced in collecting blood samples, or in starting intravenous infusions, both of which are essential duties whithin the coronary care unit. These techniques can be learned readily if the nurse spends a day or so with the hospital's laboratory technicians or "intravenous team."

Obtaining blood samples in a diabetic clinic is a similarly helpful method.

c) **Use of respiratory equipment.** Valuable practical experience in the use of positive pressure devices, manual breathing bags, mechanical respirators, and in the administration of oxygen can be obtained by having the nurse assigned for appropriate periods of time to the inhalation therapy department or to the department of anesthesiology.

d) **The technique of precordial shock.** Unquestionably the most unique experience for new nurses is the use of the defibrillator to terminate ventricular fibrillation. A machine that delivers 7,000 volts has frightening implications. Since the same method and equipment is also used to treat other, non-fatal arrhythmias (e.g., atrial fibrillation in rheumatic heart disease) on an *elective* basis, it is extremely beneficial if nurses are allowed to actually give the precordial shock in these elective cases.

After the patient has been anesthetized for the procedure, the nurse applies the paddles and delivers the shock in the physician's presence. In this way, she gains familiarity with this life-saving method and learns to use the equipment by herself when emergencies demand.

e) **Cardiopulmonary resuscitation.** It is essential that nurses be able to perform closed chest massage and "mouth-to-mouth" respiration in an effective manner. The use of life-sized mannequins (e.g., Resusci-Anne) offer an excellent method of training nurses in the techniques of cardiopulmonary resuscitation.

f) **"Fire drills" or simulated emergencies.** As a means of achieving optimal efficiency at the time of emergency situations, simulated catastrophes can be staged. Using a mannequin as a "patient" who has developed ventricular fibrillation or standstill, the nurse carries through the planned program of resuscitation, while the instructor observes the technique and times the exercise. These "fire drills" should be repeated time and again until the nurse is totally proficient.

ON–GOING EDUCATION PROGRAMS

It is important to realize that the basic training program just outlined is simply an introduction to coronary care nursing and that additional education is required if the system of coronary care is to function optimally. To this end, an on-going educational program for nurses must be developed and carried out on a continuous basis whithin each institution.

Some methods used to accomplish an effective on-going program are:

1. Team conferences

These sessions, in which all members of the coronary care unit team meet jointly, have proved to be effective and popular teaching exercises for the nursing and house staffs. The meetings consisting of case presentations and discussions of policies and practices within the unit, should be scheduled at set times once a week with the unit director presiding. These conferences provide an opportunity for mutual instruction in an informal setting and are extremely worthwhile.

The format we have employed involves a case history presentation given by a house officer (or the attending physician) after which a nurse (assigned in rotation) describes her observations about the patient's clinical course. The treatment is reviewed and special problems identified by the group.

An excerpt from one of our team conferences is reported below:

Resident physician: Mr. Scott is a 48-year-old man who was admitted to the unit yesterday afternoon following an episode of typical substernal pain along with vomiting and sweating. On admission, the pulse was 120 per minute but there were no signs of left ventricular failure. Other than the chest pain, which had persisted for an hour, his condition was quite stable. He was given 75 mg. of Demerol after which the pain disappeared. The ECG showed marked elevation of the ST segments in the precordial leads typical of acute anterior wall infarction. The rhythm showed a sinus tachycardia but no other arrhythmias. The laboratory studies showed that the CPK enzyme level was distinctly elevated. There wasn't much question about the diagnosis. I haven't seen him since late last evening but he was doing quite well then. I should add that the patient is a known diabetic who apparently has been reasonably well controlled.

Director: Dr. Edwards, as the patient's physician could you tell us a little more about his history? Did he have overt coronary disease in the past?

Attending Physician: Although this man has never had angina and an ECG six months ago was normal, I am not really surprised that he had a coronary. He would really be considered a high risk candidate. In addition to the diabetes, he smoked two packs of cigarettes a day, had an elevated serum cholesterol, and was 20 pounds overweight. Unfortunately, I was unable to get him to change his ways. Furthermore, his father died of a coronary at age 51.

Director: We would all agree this man was looking for trouble. Now, Jane, could you tell us about his course since admission?

Nurse: In general, his condition hasn't changed much during the night. He did have one other episode of chest pain about 8:00 P.M. and he was given an additional injection of Demerol. He didn't sleep well but he has not been dyspneic nor does he have any other complaints this morning. The night nurse was concerned about his pulse rate. It remained between 100 and 120 since admission and none of us has been quite sure why this sinus tachycardia has persisted.

Director: That is an important observation. We have a patient who seems stable but has a rapid heart rate. What do you make of this, John?

Resident Physician: Many patients have sinus tachycardia. It may be due to temperature elevation, anxiety, or it may reflect an early sign of impending heart failure.

Director: Quite right. What do you think is causing this patient's tachycardia?

Resident Physician: If it persisted all night and he was restless, I'd be suspicious that we may be seeing early left ventricular failure.

Nurse: That is what we guessed, too. This morning his neck veins were distended.

Director: Has a chest film been taken this morning?

Second Nurse: Yes, I called for the report just before the conference and the interpretation was early left ventricular failure.

Attending Physician: I just examined his chest and there were no rales present.

Director: That would not be unusual. The x-ray findings and the persistent tachycardia often precede clinical failure.

2. Nursing Conferences

These meetings, which represent an extension of nurse-to-nurse training, offer another means of continuous education. The conferences should be scheduled on a regular basis at such times as to enable the largest attendance without reducing nursing care in the unit. All nurse members of the team should participate in these sessions with one nurse serving as moderator in rotation. The primary purpose of nursing conferences is to permit the nursing staff to identify and seek solutions of special problems regarding patients in the coronary unit. In addition, these meetings may be used to review principles and practices of cardiac nursing, including the use and side effects of cardiac drugs; techniques of resuscitation; psychological responses of cardiac patients, etc.

An excerpt from a nursing conference follows:

Mr. Jones, a patient with acute myocardial infarction was admitted to the coronary care unit in no distress. He had no chest pain after his admission and his clinical course has been quite satisfactory. His physician has requested that Mr. Jones be kept at complete bed rest and that he be fed by the nurses. The patient has objected to this feeding and has complained bitterly to the nursing staff about this practice. The following discussion focuses on his refusal to be fed his meals.

Moderator: What reactions have you noted when you attempted to feed Mr. Jones?

Nurse No. 1: He is very unhappy. He said, "You make me feel like a baby. I feel just fine. Just let me feed myself, the doctor won't mind."

Moderator: Why do you think he has these reactions?

Nurse No. 1: For a previously active man to be fed does make him feel like a baby. He loses his manliness when submitting to being fed. Furthermore, he does not think he is ill enough for this sort of treatment.

Moderator: How do you think we can solve this problem?

Nurse No. 2: Let's ask his physician whether Mr. Jones can feed himself without causing too much exertion. If he can do this the dishes of food and the height of the tray can be positioned conveniently for him. If the doctor feels that this activity is too much we will have to explain the reasons for this limitation in more detail and offer a sympathetic, understanding attitude.

Nurse No. 3: Is this a common problem in the unit?

Moderator: It seems to be. Most patients certainly resent being fed and I wonder if this unhappiness doesn't create problems in itself.

Nurse No. 1: Why are patients fed in this way?

Nurse No. 2: Supposedly to reduce their exertion and to rest the heart but I must say this self feeding doesn't seem very vigorous to me.

Moderator: Most of our doctors seem to have abandoned the idea of "complete coronary care" and only a few of them ask that patients be fed.

Nurse No. 2: I think we ought to clarify with the doctors what they mean by "absolute rest."

Moderator: That's a good idea. I think that these rigid rules are probably outdated. We will bring this up in the team conference.

3. Ward Rounds

Because nurses working within a coronary care unit are involved with the care of patients during only one phase of the illness (i.e., the first 4-5 days) it is understandable that their view of the entire illness may become distorted. To obtain a more complete picture of acute myocardial infarction, it is important that the coronary care nurses follow the subsequent hospital course of those patients treated in the unit. This is best accomplished by having the nurses make rounds with the attending physicians throughout the hospital on a scheduled basis. In this way, the nurse can perceive the full spectrum of the hospital course of patients with acute myocardial infarction.

4. Physician Lectures

A lecture series given by several physicians during the course of the year has proven to be a valuable format for a continuing program of education. The lectures are meant to provide the nurse with an in-depth knowledge concerning various aspects of medical care as they relate to the management of patients with acute myocardial infarction.

Some representative lectures in the series might include the following subjects (and lecturers):

Respiratory therapy — Anesthesiologist

Methods of ventilation; techniques of oxygen administration; mechanical respiratory therapy; complications of artificial ventilation; blood gas studies; etc.

Emotional responses — Psychiatrist

Assessment of the patient; recognition of depression; intervening techniques; the nurses own responses; etc.

Electrocardiography — Cardiologist

Interpretation of more complex arrhythmias; electrolyte disturbances; techniques of cardiac pacing; intra-atrial electrocardiography; etc.

Pathology of myocardial infarction — Pathologist

Current concepts of atherosclerosis; significance of enzyme determinations; interpretation of results of other laboratory studies; complications of myocardial infarction; etc.

Cardiac surgery — Surgeon

Revascularization procedures; aneurysm surgery; permanent pacemaker implantation; techniques of assisted circulation; etc.

CHAPTER 6

Cardiac Monitoring

The premise of intensive coronary care had little practicality until electronic equipment was developed which was capable of measuring and displaying the electrical activity of the heart on a *continuous* basis. With these devices, known as cardiac monitors, instant detection of potentially fatal arrhythmias finally was feasible and cardiac monitoring became the cornerstone of intensive coronary care. The principles and methods of cardiac monitoring are described in this chapter.

THE CONCEPT

Each heart beat is the result of an electrical stimulus. This impulse, which normally originates in a specialized area of the heart, is then conducted through a network within the heart and finally stimulates the muscles to contract. The same electrical wave also spreads outward from the heart and reaches the surface of the body where it can be detected with electrodes attached to the skin. In this way, the heart's electrical activity can be followed continuously. This information (in the form of an electrocardiogram) is of extraordinary importance in the treatment of myocardial infarction because it permits immediate recognition of disturbances in the rate and rhythm (arrhythmia) of the heart. (The subject of electrocardiography and the interpretation of arrhythmias are considered in Chapter 9).

THE EQUIPMENT

While there are differences in the design and operation of the dozens of cardiac monitors now commercially available, their basic components and ultimate function are essentially the same.* A cardiac monitoring system works in the following way:

1) Skin electrodes, attached to the chest, pick up the electrical impulses that originate in the heart.

2) These original waves are too small to be interpreted and for this reason they are directed through an amplifier where their height is increased nearly 1,000 times.

---

* Specific advice about the selection of monitoring equipment is inappropriate here. Individual preferences will exist according to the type of coronary unit, financial considerations, and other local circumstances. However, one caution is worth noting: in purchasing equipment it is wise to select an established manufacturer who can provide for dependable, prompt service and replacement of parts at a local level.

3) The amplified impulse passes through an electrical system within the monitor where definite wave forms are established. The resultant pattern is called an *electrocardiogram.*

4) This electrocardiogram is then displayed on an oscilloscopic screen. The screen (television type) may be of different dimensions, but is usually about 5 inches or more in length.

5) Each ventricular contraction (heart beat) is counted by a rate meter which displays the average heart rate per minute. With each heart beat a sound ("beep") is audible and a light flashes.

6) Integrated with the rate meter is an alarm system which alerts the observer, by audio and visual signals, if the heart rate falls below or exceeds a pre-set level (e.g., 40-150 beats/minute). Thus, if the upper level of the alarm system is set, for example, at 150 beats per minute and the heart rate suddenly accelerates beyond this limit, the "high rate" alarm will sound.

These components fulfill the requisites for a basic monitoring system for arrhythmia detection. However, the equipment can be made more useful and elegant by the addition of other modules, including:

a) A direct write-out device to obtain a printed record of the electrocardiogram seen on the oscilloscope. This documentation can be obtained either on demand or automatically, and is valuable for comparing electrocardiographic changes.

b) A memory tape loop to record and play back the electrocardiogram of the preceding 15-60 seconds (or more). With this technique, events immediately *before* an alarm situation can be displayed subsequently if an observer was not present at the time of the occurrence.

c) Additional alarm systems that are triggered by electrocardiographic changes other than rate. These alarms may be activated by premature ventricular contractions or changes in shape of electrocardiographic waves and in this way forewarn of more serious arrhythmias.

d) Supplementary electrical circuits to indicate that a skin electrode has become disconnected or that mechanical failure exists somewhere in the monitoring system. This "lead-failure" alarm permits immediate distinction between electrical problems of instrumentation and true clinical emergencies.

PROBLEMS WITH MONITORING EQUIPMENT

It is fair to say that there is no perfect, trouble-free, monitoring system available; all monitors have certain limitations of function. While many of the difficulties encountered with earlier models have now been corrected, and new designs are constantly evolving, certain inherent problems nevertheless remain. Some of these difficulties regarding function are as follows:

The rate meter

As noted previously, this component presumably averages (and displays) the number of heart beats per minute. In fact, however, most meters are not this specific and they actually count *all* high spiked waves per minute assuming these will be the waves of ventricular contraction. Unfortunately, the contraction of skeletal muscles associated with turning in bed or moving the extremities also produce tall waves (called muscle potentials) which the rate meter is unable to distinguish from ventricular beats. It can readily be appreciated that if the device records these muscle potentials, along with actual beats, the heart rate will appear spuriously high.

The high rate alarm

Under the circumstance just described, where the rate meter misinterprets muscle potentials as heart beats (figure 3) the upper limit of the alarm system will be exceeded and a *false* alarm will result. This latter problem has been combated, to some degree by various techniques, including the "absorption" of muscle potentials by electronic filtering systems and the use of specific wave forms rather than merely the height of the waves to activate the counting mechanism of the meter. (Muscle spikes have different configurations than ventricular activity). Despite these measures, false high rate alarms are still frequent occurrences in actual practice.

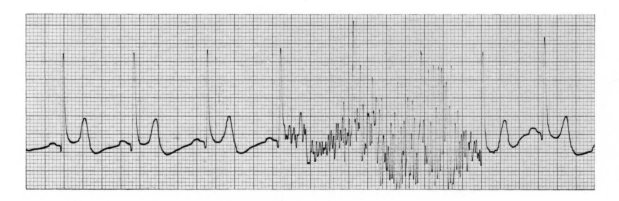

Fig. 3

The low rate alarm

The low rate alarm can be triggered falsely if contact between the electrodes and the skin becomes faulty. For example, if the electrode is not applied correctly, or if there is profuse sweating, or if the conductive paste dries, the skin-electrode contact may be disturbed. In such instances no electrical activity would be noted on the oscilloscope and it might appear as if the heart beat had stopped. The danger of mistaking this electrode failure for ventricular standstill is obvious and of serious consequence.

To prevent this problem specific "lead failure" alarms have been designed to distinguish equipment failure from lethal arrhythmias.

False low rate alarms can also occur if the R waves of the ventricular complexes are not tall enough to activate the rate meter. For example, if an arrhythmia exists where every other ventricular complex is oriented in an opposite direction to the normal beat (R) and is of reduced amplitude (see figure 4) the rate meter may not be able to detect the smaller complexes. In the electrocardiogram shown below, the true heart rate is 64 but the rate meter might record only the taller upright waves and show a rate of only 32 per minute. This would create a *false* low rate alarm.

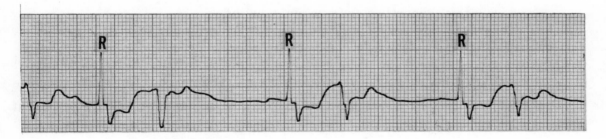

Fig. 4

Skin reactions at electrode sites

Because electrodes must remain attached to the skin for many days, inflammatory reactions at these sites are not uncommon. Proper application of the electrodes and special skin care can minimize this problem.

Distortion of electrocardiographic complexes

The electrocardiographic patterns produced by either direct write-out devices, or more particularly, by memory-tape loops, are often not true reproductions of the actual complexes as seen on the oscilloscope. This distortion results from less-than-excellent transcription modules. (Ideal reproductions from tape loops require expensive equipment that would make the total cost of the monitor unduly high). Because of these unfaithful write-outs, interpretation of arrhythmias may be difficult.

Electrical hazards

At the present time there are no uniform requirements for safety standards of electronic equipment and therefore electrical hazards may be present in certain devices. The threat of current passing accidently from the monitor to the patient, (particularly when more than one electrical system is being used) must be recognized. While efficient grounding can reduce this hazard it is important that the equipment itself be designed to prevent this risk. Unfortunately, some monitors may not be safe in this regard.

THE OPERATION OF CARDIAC MONITORS

1. Electrodes

Electrodes serve to pick up the heart's electrical signals at the surface of the skin and to transfer this current to the monitor. It is readily apparent that unless this transmission is efficient, the remaining aspects of monitoring will have little meaning; for this reason, electrodes are of great importance for succesful monitoring.

Types of Electrodes

There are 3 basic types of electrodes: 1) direct contact 2) floating, or disc type, and 3) needle electrodes. The floating electrode has become the most popular type and is used almost routinely at the present time.

1. Direct Contact Electrodes (Fig. 5)

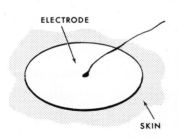

ELECTRODE

SKIN

DIRECT CONTACT ELECTRODE

These electrodes are metal plates, about 1½ inches in diameter, which resemble those used in routine electrocardiography. They are placed directly on the skin surface. A thin layer of conductive jelly (which ensures the transfer of electrical impulses) is applied at the skin-electrode interface. The electrodes are then anchored to the skin by means of adhesive or plastic tapes.

2. Floating or Disc Type Electrodes (Fig. 6)

Unlike direct contact plates, these electrodes are separated from the skin by a small built-in "spacer" which preserves a distance between the electrode and the skin. Conductive jelly fills the spacer and the electrode is attached to the skin

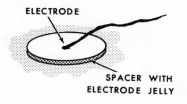

ELECTRODE

SPACER WITH
ELECTRODE JELLY

FLOATING (DISC) ELECTRODE

by an adhesive surrounding. The purpose of this separation is to reduce distortion of the heart's signal by small electrical currents existing within the skin itself. Furthermore, because the electrodes are small, electrical artifacts due to muscle potentials are reduced.

3. Needle Electrodes (Fig 7)

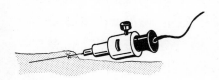

NEEDLE ELECTRODE

Small, ½ inch, 25 gauge metal-hubbed needles can be used as electrodes. These needles are inserted directly under the surface of the skin and no electrode jelly is required. With these electrodes contact is ideal, and electrical interference is minimal; furthermore, they can be placed with great rapidity in emergencies. However, these electrodes are rather difficult to keep in position and many patients find them discomforting.

Sites for Electrode Placement

To obtain the most distinct waves of ventricular activity (R waves) and thus ensure proper function of the rate meter, the electrodes should be placed in the positions shown in the following diagram.

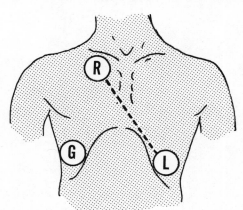

Fig. 8   **CUSTOMARY ELECTRODE POSITIONS**

The right (R) electrode is placed on the sternum medial to the right pectoral muscles. This position reduces interference from potentials arising in these muscles.

The left (L) electrode is situated at the level of the lowest palpable rib on the left side in the anterior axillary line.

The ground (G) electrode is located at a parallel site on the lower right rib cage area. This electrode simply carries off extraneous electrical currents from sources other than the heart.

With the electrode in these positions the monitor displays the electrical activity between the "R" and "L" electrodes. This particular path (or lead) normally produces the highest R waves and is chosen primarily for this reason. However, this is not uniformly true and in some cases, because of rotation of the heart or the presence of pathologic processes, the R to L lead fails to provide waves of sufficient height to activate the rate meter. In these instances another lead must be selected to obtain a greater electrical potential. This may be accomplished either by recording a different lead with the same electrode placement (e.g., the wires coming from the "R" and "G" electrodes can be switched) or by actually repositioning the electrodes at different sites.

An alternative site for electrode placement (proposed by Marriott) is shown in Fig. 9. This right chest lead produces a different wave configuration and is often useful in identifying certain arrhythmias which may not be apparent from the customary lead.

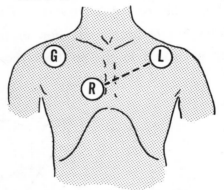

Fig. 9

RIGHT CHEST LEAD POSITIONS

Procedure for Attachment of Electrodes

Proper attachment of electrodes is undoubtedly the one most important step in cardiac monitoring. Unless there is excellent connection between the skin and the electrodes, electrical resistance will tend to distort the electrocardiographic wave form and other artifacts will appear.

1) **Prepare the designated skin areas for electrode placement.**

    a) shave chest hair in 4 inch areas around the electrode sites.

    b) clean prepared areas with a scrubbing action, using alcohol sponges. Repeat the cleansing with ether. (Unless the skin is meticulously free of oils and tissue debris the electrical impulses reaching the electrode will be affected. Painstaking care is essential for proper function).

c) allow the skin to dry thoroughly. (If sweating exists and the area does not dry, a commercial anti-perspirant spray can be used).

2) **Prepare the electrodes for use and attach to skin.**

a) Direct contact electrodes.

The metal surface of the electrode should be scrupulously clean. Cut a ¼ inch opening in a "3x3" strip of adhesive tape and insert the electrode through the slit as shown in Fig. 10.

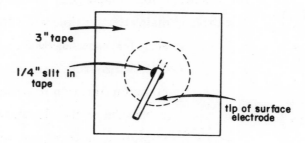

Fig. 10

Apply a small amount of electrode jelly to the skin and rub in. Additional jelly should be applied to the surface of the electrode.

Attach the electrode to the skin with the adhesive tape strip and amke certain of adhesion.

b) Floating electrodes.

Most floating electrodes are of the disposable type and the preparation for their use involves no more than removing the protecting backing which exposes a metal disc with an adhesive periphery.

A drop of electrode jelly is placed on the disc. Excessive amounts of jelly must be avoided because the conductive medium may spread and interfere with adhesion of the electrode.

The electrodes are attached firmly to the skin by manual pressure on the peripheral adhesive area and the central disc is pressed gently to insure distribution of the jelly within its structure.

c) Needle electrodes.

The needles (which must be all metal) are inserted hypodermically into the previously prepared skin sites; no electrode paste is used.

The needles are fastened in place by strips of adhesive with a technique similar to that used in securing intravenous infusions.

2. The Electrode-to-monitor Cable (The patient cable)

The signals detected by the electrodes are transmitted to the monitoring device by means of an electrical cable (the "patient" cable, in contrast to the monitor cable which goes to the wall socket for electrical supply). The cable contains the multiple wires from the individual electrodes.

Procedure for connecting cable

1) The wires from skin electrodes should be oriented in a common direction to permit their attachment to the patient cable. Unless the electrode wires are aligned in this manner stresses upon them may dislodge the skin-electrode contact.

2) The free end of each electrode wire is inserted into the designated openings of the patient cable. While these receptacles vary with different equipment each of them have clearly marked openings (often color-coded) for the respective "R," "L" and "G" electrode wires. The connectors from the electrodes must fit firmly within the cable receptacle. (Fig. 11)

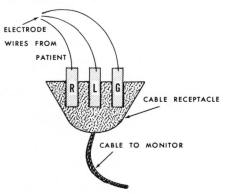

ELECTRODE WIRES FROM PATIENT

CABLE RECEPTACLE

CABLE TO MONITOR

Fig. 11   CONNECTION OF ELECTRODE WIRES

3) The monitor end of the cable is then inserted into the appropriate socket in the monitor. Again, secure contact is essential.

3. **The Monitor**

After electrode placement and connection of the cable, the monitor is ready for use. The power switch is turned "on" and the remaining components; i.e., the oscilloscope, the rate meter, and the alarm system, are then adjusted for effective function. It would be difficult to describe a uniform set of instructions for these latter procedures because of differences in design among commercially available monitors. The actual details for each of these steps are described in the manufacturer's manual of instruction which is furnished with the instrument. These guides have usually been prepared with careful thought and clearly outline the methods of operation.

Despite the differences in actual operation of various monitors a few general rules can be suggested:

1) Once the electrodes are attached, observe the electrocardiographic pattern on the oscilloscope. If the waves are of low amplitude, and cannot be increased by adjusting the sensitivity, the position of the skin electrodes should be changed to obtain a better signal or a different lead selected.

2) If there is electrical interference or if muscle potentials obscure the electrocardiographic pattern, the electrode sites should be checked carefully to ascertain if their application is correct.

3) The sensitivity dial of the monitor should be set so that *every* beat is counted by the rate meter and the audio signal (accompanying each beat) is distinct.

4) The limits of the high and low rate alarms must be set in accordance with the patient's existing heart rate and then adjusted as the clinical picture changes. Keeping the alarm limits fixed at set numbers for all patients is very poor practice.

Monitoring Problems

1) **Skin irritation**

Irritation of the chest wall is occasionally a problem with prolonged monitoring. These reactions result more often from the adhesive that secures the electrodes to the skin than from the conducting jelly or the electrodes themselves. Disposable floating electrodes can usually remain in place for several days without their position being changed. If inflammation does develop about the electrode site, the area should be treated with an emollient or anesthetic cream and the electrode repositioned a few inches away.

If direct contact electrodes are used, it is advisable to remove these metal plates once a day and to clean the skin sites with soap and water before reapplying them.

2) **Electrocardiographic signals of poor quality.**

Indistinct or defective patterns seen on the oscilloscope may result from several causes including poor contact of electrodes, improper connection of the patient cable, or malfunction of the monitoring device. Without question, the most common source of poor oscilloscopic patterns is faulty contact between the electrode and the skin. Therefore, the first step in determining why a signal is unsatisfactory involves a deliberate examination of the electrode contact. Typical problems which may disturb this contact are: improper attachment of the electrode to the skin; inadequate (or sometimes too much) conductive jelly; or profuse sweating. All of these result in some displacement.

3) **Electrical Interference.**

In some coronary care units electrical current from other sources (power lines, other electronic equipment, etc.) creates interference with the monitor signal. While the equipment itself is grounded to combat this problem and a separate ground ("G") electrode is also used to carry off extraneous electrical activity, interference of this type is nevertheless a common disturbance. If this problem persists, additional grounding circuits within the unit may be needed.

4) **False alarms**

For reasons previously described, false high and low rate alarms can and do occur during the course of monitoring. In order to minimize the annoyance of these false alarms there is a temptation to set the alarm limits widely apart (e.g., 40-180 rather than 60-110), or still worse, to run the alarm system off when false alarms are frequent. This practice renders the system useless and should never be adopted.

CHAPTER 7

Coronary Care Nursing
The Nursing Role in the Admission
of Patients and in their Subsequent Care

In the final analysis intensive coronary care is an advanced system of nursing. The number of lives saved with this specialized care can be directly related to the competence of the nurses in the coronary unit.

To clearly define this nursing role it is appropriate to first outline the total duties and responsibilities of the CCU nurse and then to consider specific nursing care procedures that are followed from the time of admission to discharge.

AN OUTLINE OF NURSING DUTIES AND RESPONSIBILITIES

1. **Continuous Assessment of the Patient's Cardiac Status**

    a. With the Use of Monitoring Equipment

    The nurse must be aware of the heart rhythm at all times and be able to distinguish all significant arrhythmias. This ability requires a usable knowledge of electrocardiography and an understanding of the principles and operation of monitoring devices. Much of the success of the coronary care system is dependent on this nursing duty.

    b. By Repeated Direct Observation of the Patient

    Because monitors offer information about only one aspect of the heart, namely, its electrical activity, the remaining phases of cardiac performance must be assessed by other means. In particular, to evaluate the heart's function as a pump a series of planned observations at the bedside must be made. To this end, the nurse deliberately and carefully seeks various signs and symptoms which may reflect decreased mechanical function of the heart.

2. **Special duties relating to treatment**

    A coronary care unit nurse must be able to perform the following therapeutic measures at her own discretion without specific orders.*

---

* Because the coronary care unit nurse is delegated with responsibilities that transcend usual duties of nurses, it is worthwhile to establish a series of policies which authorize the nurse to utilize her judgement in the management of certain problems. These policies should be clearly described in written form so that all concerned are in agreement about this delegation of authority to the nurse. Many hospitals prefer to include these policies in the form of a prepared order, signed by the attending physician.

a) Administer oxygen by a method appropriate for the clinical situation.

b) Start intravenous infusions.

c) Anticipate the treatment program and prepare drugs for each emergency situation. (In many coronary care units nurses are authorized to administer certain antiarrhythmic drugs, such as lidocaine or atropine, on the basis of their clinical judgement).

d) Terminate ventricular fibrillation by precordial shock (defibrillation) in the absence of the physician.

e) Perform cardiopulmonary resuscitation.

f) Apply and rotate tourniquets in the treatment of left ventricular failure.

g) Use equipment for respiratory assistance, including mechanical respirators and manual breathing bags.

3. Routine Nursing Care

In addition to her specialized duties, the coronary care unit nurse gives general nursing care to the patients in the unit. The plan of nursing care for the coronary patient must have great flexibility. Instead of establishing rigid routines for nursing measures, only general policies should be developed which permit the plan to be altered according to individual needs.

4. Laboratory studies

To minimize confusion resulting from multiple hospital personnel within the unit and to preserve serenity, the coronary care unit nurse should be able to perform the following laboratory procedures:

a) Record a 12 lead electrocardiogram.

b) Collect blood samples for laboratory determinations.

c) Organize laboratory results in an orderly way so that variations in serial determinations are readily apparent to the team members.

5. Emotional support

The nurse should identify the emotional reactions of patients in the coronary unit by thoughtful interpretation of verbal and non-verbal clues. On this basis, she should attempt to provide necessary emotional support to these critically ill patients.

6. Communication

As a member of the coronary care team the nurse must communicate with the patient, his family, as well as her colleagues. The main duties in this regard are:

a) To explain the concept of coronary care to the patient and his family in order to allay their fears and to obtain their co-operation.

b) To serve as a liaison between the physician, the patient, and his family.

c) To advise the physician directly of meaningful changes in the patient's status.

d) To present a succinct and comprehensive report to the other members of the nursing staff.

7. **Data collection and recording**

The nurse should obtain and record pertinent information relative to variations in the patient's clinical condition. These data should include:

a) Rhythm strips of electorcardiogram to document arrhythmias.

b) Changes in signs or symptoms.

c) Drug therapy, including time of administration and effect.

d) Other therapeutic measures.

e) Emotional responses.

8. **Teaching**

The experienced coronary care nurse should serve as a preceptor for new nurses joining the coronary care team.

THE PATIENT WHO IS NOT IN ACUTE DISTRESS ON ADMISSION

1. **Connect chest electrode and initiate cardiac monitoring.**

Since arrhythmias may develop at any time, and particularly in the immediate hours after infarction, it is essential that electrocardiographic monitoring be started as soon as the patient is admitted. This measure should be the *first step* in the care of the patient regardless of his clinical condition.

2. **Explain the monitoring system to the patient and describe the general program of care within the coronary unit.**

It should be appreciated that the procedure of continuous monitoring will be unfamiliar to most patients, and may be frightening to them. For this reason, and because patient co-operation will be needed for effective care, it is important that the nurse briefly but clearly explain the monitoring system and the concept of coronary care to the patient at this time. A taped interview of a nurse giving this information is found on page 75.

3. **Record an electrocardiographic strip to document the cardiac rhythm.**

This initial rhythm strip has significant implications in terms of the treatment program and the overall prognosis. Because it serves as a base line for future comparison, the rhythm strip should be taken as early after admission as possible. The strip should then be stapled to the nurse's admission records.

4. **Inquire about the presence of chest pain.**

It is a basic rule of therapy in acute myocardial infarction to control chest pain promptly. Ischemic pain is usually a source of great apprehension to the patient and relief of this distressing symptom should be accomplished without delay. If the patient complains of chest pain, the nurse should administer a narcotic as ordered by the physician.

5. **Assess the patient's clinical status and record pertinent information.**

The major aim at the time of admission is to determine whether the patient has signs or symptoms of cardiac failure or cardiogenic shock. In addition, the presence of pre-existing diseases which may influence the course of treatment should be ascertained. This information should be recorded on the nurse's admission summary sheet. (see page 79).

6. **Start an intravenous infusion.**

It is customary practice in most coronary units to establish and maintain an intravenous line for all patients with acute myocardial infarction. This "keep-open" intravenous pathway eliminates the waste of precious time in administering intravenous drugs in emergency situations. The nurse should start an infusion containing 5% glucose in water for this purpose.

7. **Notify the physician.**

The nurse should communicate her findings to the physician responsible for the patient's immediate care (i.e., the attending physician or a house officer). This verbal report should summarize the clinical and electrocardiographic status at the time of admission. Appropriate arrangements should be made regarding the initial phases of the treatment program.

8. **Record a 12 lead electrocardiogram.**

This tracing is important for comparative purposes in establishing the diagnosis of acute myocardial infarction. (If a 12 lead tracing has been taken in the physician's office or in the receiving ward shortly before admission to the unit it is not necessary to repeat the ECG at this time).

9. **Collect blood and urine samples for laboratory determinations.**

To minimize patient anxiety and for the sake of expediency, the nurse, rather than a technician, should collect appropriate blood and urine specimens for laboratory study. Most hospitals have established a routine set of studies for all patients at the time of admission to the coronary care unit.

10. **Assist the physician in the physical examination of the patient.**

The nurse should compare the findings and impressions of the physician with those she made originally. Variations in the blood pressure, pulse rate, cardiac rhythm and other clinical observations occurring in the interval may be extremely important in determining the treatment program.

11. **Begin the treatment program as ordered by the physician.**

The proposed management of the patient should be discussed in detail with the physician so that the nurse has a clear picture of the aims of therapy and problems that may be anticipated. Drug therapy should be started promptly and the time of administration carefully recorded.

12. **Arrange for other studies.**

Studies, including radiographic examination of the chest and measurement of central venous pressure, are commonly (or routinely) performed in many institutions. The nurse should arrange for, and assist in these procedures.

13. **Explain the situation to the family.**

The obvious concern of families for these dangerously ill patients must be fully appreciated, as well as the fact that the patient is one of the family and cannot be set apart simply because he is in the hospital. With this in mind, the nurse should give a general description of the unit and its purpose to the family visitors and reassure them. It is unwise to view the family as burdensome; their cooperation should be enlisted. This situation is well handled by a nurse in the taped interview on page 76.

14. **Allay the patient's fears.**

After these initial procedures have been completed, the nurse should spend some time simply talking to the patient. The emotional trauma with a myocardial infarction is often profound and the fear of sudden death is frequently expressed. It is of major importance to offer strong support to the patient at this time.

THE PATIENT WHO IS IN ACUTE DISTRESS ON ADMISSION

1. **Connect the electrodes and obtain a rhythm strip.**

The incidence of lethal arrhythmias is unusually high in the presence of shock or left ventricular failure and the monitoring system should be put into operation before anything else is attempted. Since most deaths that occur within the first 30 minutes after admission are due to arrhythmias, preparations for these sudden catastrophes should precede other therapy.

2. **Notify the physician immediately.**

Patients admitted in acute distress undoubtedly have developed a serious complication of acute myocardial infarction (most likely left ventricular failure, cardiogenic shock, or a profound rhythm disturbance) and therapy must be started as soon as possible. The earlier treatment is initiated in these critical circumstances, the better the chances for survival. For this reason, the nurse should advice the physician of the patient's status at once.

3. **Start oxygen therapy.**

Oxygen should be administered without delay in all acutely ill patients. The most effective method for delivering oxygen in this situation involves the use of a tight fitting face mask with a flow rate of 8-10 liters of oxygen per minute.

4. **Start an intravenous infusion.**

Because intravenous drug therapy will be used in the treatment program an intravenous conduit should be established as soon as practicable; this infusion should contain 5% of glucose in water.

5. **Assess the patient's clinical condition and record the findings.**

The blood pressure, pulse rate, number and quality of respiration, color of the skin, presence or absence of sweating, mental status, urinary output, as well as electrocardiographic findings should be carefully noted and recorded. These data allow meaningful comparisons.

6. **Prepare for emergency treatment program.**

   Equipment and drugs to be used in the treatment of the complication should be brought to the bedside and prepared for immediate use.

7. **Start the treatment program as ordered by the physician, or in accordance with the standard procedure of the coronary care unit.**

   Having identified the complication which created the acute distress, a *planned* program to combat the problem should be instituted by the coronary care team. The nursing role in the treatment of left ventricular failure, cardiogenic shock, and arrhythmias is described in detail in subsequent chapters.

THE NURSING ROLE IN THE SUBSEQUENT CARE OF PATIENTS

From hour to hour the nurse may be faced with a variety of problems that must be resolved as they occur. She has to make prompt decisions about whether to observe the course of clinical or electrocardiographic changes by herself, or to call a physician, or to initiate emergency treatment without delay. Decisions of this sort require sound judgement which can only be acquired by combining good training with experience.

In addition to these specialized duties relative to the cardiac status, the nurse has the fundamental responsibility (common to all good nursing practice) of identifying and meeting other individual needs of patients. In making decisions it is essential that the nurse view the patient as a whole and not confine her attention only to the monitor and the cardiovascular system.

Bedside nursing is still vital to good care. The presence of monitors and other elaborate equipment does not relieve the nurse of this basic duty. In effect, equipment complements rather than supplements nursing care.

General nursing care during the course of a day is flexible. The nurse plans and implements her care according to needs of the individual patient and the circumstances. Therefore, if the patient is sleeping, she postpones nursing measures until a later time; or if blood samples are needed for chemistry determinations, she performs the procedure at a convenient rather than a set time.

The following outline is a guide to aspects of general nursing care within a coronary unit.

Direct Patient Care

Routine care of the cardiac patient includes these measures:

1. Check the vital signs (temperature, pulse, respirations, and blood pressure) at intervals commensurate with the patient's clinical status.

Unless these findings are compared deliberately with those made previously, their value is markedly reduced.

2. Assess fluid and electrolyte balance by carefully recording the intake and output of fluids. This information is often of great importance in the management of patients, and the nurse must recognize the need for wholly accurate data in this regard. The duty should not be minimized by its delegation to untrained personnel.

3. Maintain body hygiene (with its attendant physical comfort) through periodic cleansing. As noted, the nurse should use her discretion in planning when baths and other hygienic measures are to be given; rigid schedules must be avoided.

4. Position the patient to assure his comfort. While semi-Fowler's position is customary for patients with acute myocardial infarction (to allow for adequate lung expansion) this position can, and should be, varied several times each shift.

5. Facilitate elimination by assisting the patient in the use of a bedside commode. The use of bedpans has fallen into disfavor because of the high expenditure of energy involved and the awkwardness of its use. Stool softening drugs and mild cathartics are sensible additions to this problem.

6. Evaluate the adequacy of nutrition and assist the patient achieving a proper and sensible diet. Because sodium restriction is a common practice in this setting, many patients find their diets unpalatable. The nurse should recognize this problem and attempt to make food more attractive by using flavors such as lemon, thyme, vinegar, and other sodium free spices.

7. Maintain optimal body mechanics with passive exercises. The extremities should be moved through their full range of motion several times a day.

8. Provide a restful environment within the coronary care unit by limiting the number of visitors and by controlling noise and confusion.

9. Administer medications and carefully observe the response in terms of desired effects and possible side effects.

10. Control the patient's physical activity to minimize the work load of the heart.

Psychological Support of the Patient

Many patients who sustain an acute myocardial infarction develop an intense emotional response. This psychological reaction is understandable since patients are usually aware that the attack may threaten their lives in many ways. Unfortunately, the impact on the patient is frequently intensified by the very nature of the specialized care he is given. The system of coronary care involving constant monitoring, continuous surveillance, intravenous infusions, and repeated examinations and studies within a confined and busy setting may create obvious anxiety.

Recognizing these threats along with the fact that the patient has suddenly become completely dependent, it becomes clear that psychological support is an essential part of the treatment program. The nursing role in this regard is of fundamental importance.

There are several ways that the nurse can assist the patient to adjust to this stressful situation:

1. Encourage him to express his feelings. By listening attentively and evincing genuine interest, the nurse can assist the patient to ventilate his fears. This form of emotional support is of great help in most patients.

2. Offer reassurance. By acting in a calm, positive, organized and efficient manner, the coronary care team instills confidence among the patients in the unit. In many ways this truly professional demeanor represents the most effective means of reassurance.

3. Answer questions in a forthright manner. If a patient asks the nurse a specific question about his illness, the inquiry should be answered directly. By avoiding the question or by simply saying, "You will have to ask the doctor," the nurse may indirectly intensify the patient's anxiety.

4. Explain the equipment, procedures, and the reasons for various measures employed in the treatment program.

5. Discuss rehabilitation. Because of the excellent rapport that often develops between the CCU nurses and the patient, there is a unique opportunity to offer valuable assistance in the eventual rehabilitation of the patient. Among patients who are not acutely ill, this program can be initiated during the early days in the unit. However, if this is not feasible during the first few days, the nurse can visit the patient after his transfer elsewhere in the hospital and pursue this goal. The basic theme in rehabilitation is to offer a hopeful outlook and to make the patient aware that he can lead a useful, productive life despite the myocardial infarction. It should be stressed that normal activities are beneficial

rather than dangerous. It is particularly important to explain the heart's ability to develop collateral circulation which, in effect, may serve as the equivalent of a new blood supply to replace the occluded vessels.

THE NURSING ROLE IN THE TRANSFER OF PATIENTS FROM CCU

Unless patients are to receive intensive coronary care throughout the entire period of hospitalization (a problem considered previously), preparation must be made for the transfer of patients from the protected atmosphere of the unit to regular hospital facilities. In some instances, this poses no difficulties and the nurse simply indicates to the patient that his improvement is such that intensive care is no longer needed and that in the next day or so he will be transferred from the unit. In other cases this transition is more difficult because of the patient's dependency on constant nursing care and the equipment. Here, the nurse must convince the patient of the safety of this move and offer repeated reassurance in order to minimize anxiety and fear. The nurse should carefully evaluate the patient's emotional response to the proposed transfer and use her discretion and judgement in handling this matter. When an untoward emotional reaction seems evident, a cooperative effort by all members of the nursing care team can avert difficult (a method of handling this problem appears on page 77 and 78).

TAPED INTERVIEW BETWEEN NURSE AND PATIENT EXPLAINING THE MONITORING SYSTEM AND THE PROGRAM OF CARE

Nurse: I am going to attach these electrodes to your chest, Mr. Clark. This won't bother you a bit.

Patient: Is this another heart test?

Nurse: No, this isn't a test. The purpose of these electrodes is to allow us to watch your heart beat while you are here in the unit. Every time the heart beats it sends out an electrical signal and these little electrodes pick up the signal and send it along to the monitor in the nursing station. In this way, we can tell how your heart is beating all the time.

Patient: I must be in pretty bad shape if you have to do all that!

Nurse: Oh, no, you are not in bad shape. We monitor every patient in the unit. By knowing the condition of your heart every second we are able to pick up the first sign of any trouble that may be developing. The whole idea of this monitoring is to *prevent* trouble.

Patient: Will I be able to move around with all these electrodes and wires?

Nurse: Yes. You can forget all about them once I have them all attached. Of course, we don't want the electrodes to come loose, or the wires to be disconnected so you have to be careful about this.

Patient: Do you disconnect them every time I want to go to the bathroom?

Nurse: No, the electrodes have to remain in place all the time otherwise we wouldn't be able to follow your heart beat. Besides, you are going to have to remain pretty much at complete bed rest for the next few days and you will use a commode we bring to the bedside when you need it.

Patient: Are you sure I'm not pretty sick? This seems like a lot with all these wires and not being able to get out of bed.

Nurse: As Dr. Thompson told you, he believes that you have had a heart attack. You remember he said that one of the pipe lines to the heart muscle has blocked off and that part of the muscle is injured. It is just like any other injury - in order to get it to heal the part must be rested. That's why you must be at bed rest for the next several days. Rest allows the heart to heal.

Patient: How long does it take to heal?

Nurse: It depends on many things and varies in different people. You will probably be in this unit for about 4 or 5 days and then you will be transferred to a regular hospital room.

Patient: What else happens to me while I'm in this unit?

Nurse: Other than being monitored the nurses and doctors are going to keep a very close watch on how your heart is behaving. As I said our main job here is to prevent trouble and that's just what we will be doing. In fact, this intravenous fluid I am about to start is part of this program of prevention. We are going to keep this dripping very slowly so that we can give you any medications you may need immediately if we saw some change on the monitor.

Patient: I guess I don't have much choice.

Nurse: All of this isn't going to be as unpleasant as you think. I'll tell you more about it when I come back in a little while.

TAPED INTERVIEW BETWEEN NURSE AND FAMILY VISITOR EXPLAINING THE MONITORING SYSTEM AND THE CCU PROGRAM

Nurse: Mrs. Taylor, I am Miss Smith. Your husband is doing fine and we will let you visit him just as soon as his studies are finished.

Patient's wife: Oh, thank God! I was so worried when they called me at home. What has happened to him?

Nurse: The doctor believes your husband has had a heart attack. It means that one of the arteries that bring blood to the heart muscle is blocked off and a portion of the heart has been injured.

Patient's wife: Isn't that terribly serious?

Nurse: The heart can heal very well. The main job right now is to prevent any complications from developing and it is for this reason that your husband has been admitted to this special unit called the Coronary Care Unit. It is only for patients with heart attacks.

Patient's wife: I think I read about this special care in the newspaper. It is an electronic machine isn't it?

Nurse: Part of his care does involve a cardiac monitor but the most important thing is that he will be observed continuously by a trained team of nurses and doctors. Let me show you the monitoring system. (The nurse explains the function of the monitor).

Patient's wife: This is just wonderful! Is there a doctor here all the time in case something shows on the monitor?

Nurse: No, it is the nurse's job to watch the monitor and to look for signs of trouble. All of us have been specially trained for this work, and one or more of us are here every minute of the day and night. If we see any changes in a patient's condition we report this immediately to the doctor.

Patient's wife: I feel so relieved. Can I visit him any time or are there special hours?

Nurse: Here is a little folder which tells about visiting hours, phone calls, and that sort of thing. If you have any questions we will be glad to help you.

Patient's wife: How long will my husband be in the unit?

Nurse: Most of our patients stay in the unit for about five days but the time varies. The doctor will keep you advised of his plans.

TAPED INTERVIEW BETWEEN NURSE AND PATIENT REGARDING TRANSFER FROM THE CCU

Nurse: Dr. Cohen just told me the good news. I understand you are going to be transferred from our unit tomorrow.

Patient: That's what he told me but I just wonder if I should not spend a few more days here.

Nurse: You must like it here very much. Only a few days ago you were unhappy about coming to the unit and now you don't want to leave.

Patient: Well I'm just a little concerned what might happen if my heart changed suddenly and nobody was around at the time. They don't monitor you in regular rooms, do they?

Nurse: No, you will not be monitored once you leave the unit. In fact, it is because you don't need monitoring any longer that Dr. Cohen is transferring you.

Patient: How does he know that my heart won't act up once I am out of here?

Nurse: He knows that you have already passed the danger period and that it is quite safe to move you.

Patient: I'm glad to hear that but I still don't like the idea of being all alone.

Nurse: You are not going to be all alone. There are always nurses nearby and you will still have the same doctor. Besides, we will come and visit you and say hello. The only big difference after your transfer will be no more machines and nurses peeking at you all day. That should be a pleasant relief.

Patient: That's one way to look at it.

NURSE'S ADMISSION SUMMARY

Name _Elliott, John_   Age _51_   Sex _M_

Date & Hour of Admission _5/12/70 — 2:30 P.M._

Attending Physician _Thomas Scott, M.D._ Admitting Nurse _K. Davies, R.N._

Past History

previous infarction _no_
known diabetes _yes_
other known diseases _hypertension — 5 yrs._
previous medications _Orinase tab ī bid_
Diural 500 mg. daily

Symptoms on Admission

chest pain _yes, moderately severe pain relieved ī 100 mg. Demerol_
dyspnea _mild, improved ī oxygen by nasal cannula._

Physical findings on Admission

blood pressure _158/98_
pulse rate _112_
temperature _98⁶_
skin _dry, no sweating_

Cardiac rhythm _Sinus tachycardia. No PVCˢ_
(staple rhythm strip to
back of this sheet)

Summary of clinical condition _Admitted ī chest pain and mild dyspnea but not in acute distress._

Laboratory Studies	Ordered	Performed	Nursing Comment
CBC	✓		
Urinalysis	✓	✓	
BUN	✓	✓	Clinitest: 2+ glucose, trace acetone
Blood Sugar (2 hrs. p.p.)	✓	✓	stat sugar — 222 mg.%
CPK	✓	✓	
SGOT	✓	✓	
Sed. rate	✓	✓	
Prothrombin time	NO	—	
Lee white time	NO	—	
ECG (12 lead)	✓	✓	
Chest x-ray	✓	✓	

The Major Complications of Acute Myocardial Infarction and the Related Nursing Role

There are 5 major complications of acute myocardial infarction:

Acute Heart Failure

Cardiogenic Shock

Thromboembolism

Ventricular rupture

and

Cardiac Arrhythmias

It is essential to realize that deaths following acute myocardial infarction are due to one or more of these complications. It is only by the prevention of complications, or successful treatment of these problems that lives can be saved. This is the very theme of intensive coronary care.

ACUTE HEART FAILURE

In the interval between contractions (diastole) both ventricles promptly fill with blood from their respective venous systems. With the next ventricular beat (systole) this volume of blood is expelled into the arterial tree. If for some reason the ventricles become unable to empty completely with each contraction, the heart is said to be in *failure*. The blood remaining in the ventricle tends to impede the subsequent venous return and an elevation in venous pressure gradually develops. This creates, in effect, a back flow of blood into the atria and venous channels.

The heart attempts to compensate for this problem by increasing its rate and the force of contractions. In this way adequate circulation may continue, at least temporarily, until these compensatory mechanisms are no longer effective. At this point (decompensation) there are distinctive signs and symptoms of acute heart failure. If the condition is not corrected the total circulation ultimately fails and the vital tissues become deprived of oxygen. As a result of this anoxemia irreversible arrhythmias occur and death follows.

Acute heart failure may develop immediately after the infarction or over a period of days or weeks depending on several factors including the extent of myocardial damage and the ability of the heart to compensate for its inefficiency.

To understand the clinical course and treatment of acute heart failure, it is essential to consider the heart as two separate pumping systems, with the right heart as the pump for the pulmonary circulation and the left heart as the driving force for the systemic circulation (Fig. 12).

Because myocardial infarction involves the left ventricle almost exclusively it is understandable that *left heart failure* is by far the more common form of decompensation in this situation. *Right heart failure* is almost always secondary to left heart failure in patients with acute myocardial infarction and seldom exists independently.

LEFT HEART FAILURE

Because of either tissue destruction resulting from the infarction or metabolic changes in the myocardium secondary to ischemia, the left ventricle is weakened and its pumping ability is reduced. This reduction in ventricular efficiency results in a decrease in the volume of blood ejected with each contraction (the *stroke volume)*. In turn, the total volume of blood pumped per minute (the *cardiac output*) falls. This diminution in cardiac output may be modest or profound and the clinical picture of left ventricular failure in a sense reflects the extent of this particular hemodynamic deficit.

When the left ventricle fails, it loses its ability to empty completely with each contraction. As a result, the flow of blood returning from the lungs to the incompletely emptied ventricle is impeded and a back pressure develops in the left atrium and in turn the pulmonary veins. The engorged veins tend to impose on the available air space within the lung, but more significantly, the increased venous pressure forces fluid from the pulmonary capillary system into the lung tissues causing *pulmonary edema*. This exudation of fluid into the lungs produces the clinical state described as *acute left ventricular failure*. The spectrum of left ventricular failure has several degrees of intensity.

The Clinical Spectrum of Left Ventricular Failure

1. **Subclinical or incipient left ventricular failure**

    The *initial* effect of reduced left ventricular function is an increase in the pressure within the pulmonary veins, as already noted. At its onset this pulmonary venous hypertension does *not* produce either symptoms or clinical signs, and is therefore designated as *subclinical* failure. The presence of this first manifestation of left ventricular failure can be detected, however, by x-ray examination of the chest. The classical radiographic finding indicative of increased pulmonary venous pressure is dilatation of the pulmonary veins in the upper lobes of the lungs.(Fig. 13).

CIRCULATION THROUGH LEFT AND RIGHT HEART
Schematic Diagram

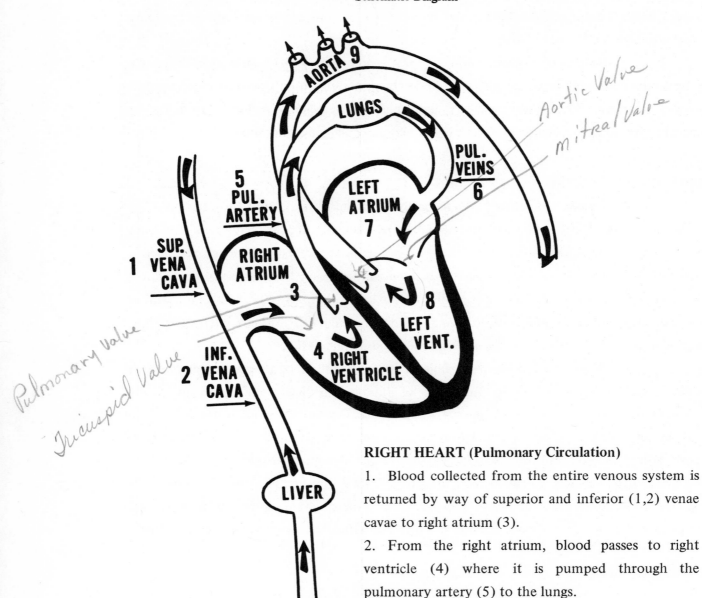

Fig. 12

RIGHT HEART (Pulmonary Circulation)

1. Blood collected from the entire venous system is returned by way of superior and inferior (1,2) venae cavae to right atrium (3).

2. From the right atrium, blood passes to right ventricle (4) where it is pumped through the pulmonary artery (5) to the lungs.

3. In the lungs, carbon dioxide is removed from the blood, and oxygenated blood returns by way of the pulmonary veins (6) to the left heart.

LEFT HEART (Systemic Circulation)

1. Oxygenated blood from the pulmonary veins enters the left atrium (7) and passes to the left ventricle (8).

2. Contraction of the left ventricle propels the blood through the aorta (9) and to the systemic circulation.

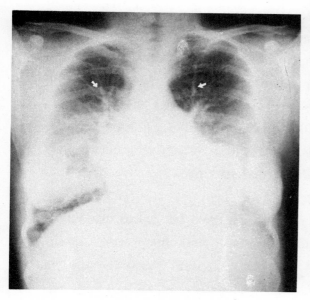

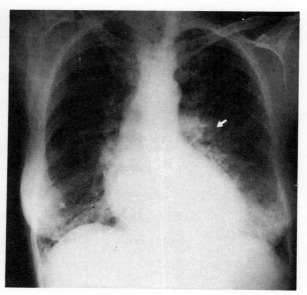

Fig. 13   Fig. 14

If the pulmonary venous pressure continues to rise, small amounts of fluid are forced through the capillary walls into the interstitial tissues which surround the air cells (alveoli) of the lung. This collection of fluid is described as *interstitial edema*. It represents a progression of pulmonary venous hypertension. This stage of left ventricular failure is also subclinical and does not produce dyspnea nor can it be detected by physical examination; but its presence can be clearly noted, in most instances, on the chest x-ray (Fig 14).

It is believed (but not fully proven) that by detecting and treating left ventricular failure in these incipient stages that the progress to more advanced left ventricular failure can be halted. It is on this basis that x-ray examination of the chest has become a standard procedure in many coronary care units.

2.   Clinical or overt left ventricular failure

When left ventricular failure progresses additionally, edema fluid is forced into the alveoli themselves; this collection of fluid within the air spaces is called *alveolar edema*. Such edema distinctly reduces oxygen and carbon dioxide exchange and *dyspnea* usually occurs as a consequence.

Alveolar edema, unlike interstitial edema, is clearly evident on physical examination by the presence of rales at the bases of the lungs. This single finding identifies *overt* left ventricular failure and is a definite indication to start a treatment program to combat heart failure.

A second classical sign of left heart failure is the detection of a *gallop rhythm* on stethoscopic examination. Normally, the heart has two distinct sounds designated simply as the first and second heart sounds. When the left ventricle fails, a third heart sound is frequently heard. Because the cadence of the three sounds resembles the sound of a galloping horse the rhythm is descriptively termed a gallop rhythm. The presence of a gallop rhythm is a cardinal sign of left ventricular failure whether or not rales are identified at the same time.

3. **Paroxysmal Nocturnal Dyspnea**

For reasons that are not wholly clear, marked left ventricular failure sometimes develops with seeming abruptness while the patient is asleep; hence the name *paroxysmal nocturnal dyspnea.* These episodes of sudden dyspnea represent acute decompensation of the left ventricle. The usual clinical story of paroxysmal nocturnal dyspnea is that about 1-2 hours after falling asleep the patiend awakens *suddenly* with marked dyspnea. He complains of suffocation and great fear is usually evident. Paroxysms of coughing often accompany the dyspnea. Breathing is usually improved in the sitting position and most patients assume this posture promptly or leave the bed and attempt to reach a nearby window, believing that fresh air will help their breathing. The attack may subside within a few minutes in a sitting position or the episode may worsen progressively with dyspnea and coughing becoming more severe. Although paroxysmal nocturnal dyspnea usually occurs with dramatic suddeness, it is quite likely that left ventricular failure existed previously in a subclinical stage and that the progression was insidious.

4. **Acute Pulmonary Edema**

The most advanced stage of acute left heart failure is *pulmonary edema.* It is akin to paroxysmal nocturnal dyspnea in etiology and treatment but differs in the sense that it need not begin suddenly in the recumbent position and usually represents a progression or culmination of earlier signs of failure. Unlike paroxysmal nocturnal dyspnea which may end spontaneously, acute pulmonary edema is generally continuous and must be treated vigorously.

The clinical picture of acute pulmonary edema is distinctive and usually poses no problem in diagnosis. Dyspnea is profound and cyanosis may be present. Gurgling sounds are audible from the respiratory tree and coughing is most often incessant. The sputum is typically frothy and may be blood tinged. In conjunction with these signs of obvious respiratory difficulty, the pulse rate is rapid, and profuse sweating is usually observed; there can be little doubt that the patient is in acute distress.

The Treatment of Left Ventricular Failure

There are three fundamental objectives in the overall treatment program:

1) To improve the performance and function of the left ventricle. This is accomplished primarily by the use of digitalis.

2) to lessen the workload of the failing left ventricle by reducing the volume of blood returning to it. Measures employed for this purpose include diuretics, tourniquets and phlebotomy.

3) to improve tissue oxygenation so that adequate perfusion can be maintained during the period of failure.

The actual sequence of treatment and the methods used depends fundamentally on the degree of left ventricular failure. The treatment of acute pulmonary edema is of most concern and is described in the following paragraphs.

The Treatment of Acute Pulmonary Edema

1) Morphine is used immediately and should precede all other forms of therapy. Not only does this narcotic combat the distressing anxiety associated with acute pulmonary edema but more significantly it depresses the respiratory centers in the brain and reduces the number of respirations. By slowing respiration in this way the volume of blood returning from the lungs to the left ventricle is reduced.

2) Oxygen therapy is of particular importance during the period of respiratory embarrassment. As a result of marked alveolar edema it is readily understandable that the concentration of oxygen in the blood may be drastically reduced. As a consequence, oxygen must be administered to preserve tissue function. A tight-fitting face mask is probably the most efficient means of delivering oxygen in this situation; nasal cannulae are much less desirable. Some physicians prefer to administer oxygen with positive pressure devices in this acute setting.

3) Rapid acting diuretics, such as furosemide (Lasix), or ethacrynic acid (Edecrin) administered intravenously usually produce dramatic improvement within minutes; dyspnea abates promptly and there is a voluminous diuresis. Theoretically these agents are effective because

they induce excretion of extracellular fluid and therefore reduce the volume of blood returning to the left ventricle. However, the extraordinary rapidity with which pulmonary edema is controlled by these drugs suggests that a more complicated pharmacologic mechanism of action is operative.

4) Digitalis is extremely valuable in this acute emergency. Unlike morphine or diuretic therapy which tend to decrease venous return to the left ventricle, digitalis directly improves the pumping action of the failing ventricle. On this basis, digitalis is essential to restoring adequate cardiac function. In this desperate situation the most rapid-acting digitalis preparations are preferable (e.g., Cedilanid, ouabain or digoxin) and should be administered intravenously.

5) **Other methods of treatment**

In the event that morphine, diuretics and digitalis are not immediately successful, the use of rotating tourniquets can be attempted. By trapping venous blood in the extremities with the tourniquets, the circulating blood can be reduced. This technique, while popular in the past, has assumed much less importance since the introduction of the very effective rapid-acting diuretics.

The blood volume can also be reduced promptly by means of phlebotomy during which 500 cc. or more is withdrawn from the body into a vaccum-type container. This method is used only if other means have failed and is seldom required.

RIGHT HEART FAILURE

In acute myocardial infarction the right heart fails, in most instances, as a sequel to left heart failure; isolated right heart failure is extremely rare. This relationship between left and right heart failure can be viewed as follows: when the left heart fails, significant back pressure develops in the pulmonary veins and capillaries, as already noted. Blood, being pumped from the *right* ventricle through the pulmonary arteries, therefore meets ultimate resistance in the pulmonary capillaries causing the pressure to rise in the main pulmonary artery. As the pulmonary artery pressure mounts, the right ventricle becomes unable to empty completely with each contraction. The residual volume of blood within this ventricle then impedes the emptying of the right atrium. As a consequence blood returning from the superior and inferior vena cavae meets resistance. This creates a back pressure throughout the entire peripheral venous system leading to engorgement or congestion of the venous tree. The resulting clinical picture is called *congestive* heart failure.

While this etiologic concept, called *backward* heart failure, is logical and explains many of the typical findings of right heart failure, it is quite certain that the problem of the failing heart is infinitely more complicated. For instance, it is well known that congestive heart failure is accompanied by the retention of sodium and water, and that renal function is disturbed. These latter changes cannot fully be explained simply by increased back pressure and it is apparent that renal and hormonal factors (e.g., aldosterone) also contribute to the total picture of right heart failure. It is believed that the decreased cardiac output and other hemodynamic derangements that accompany heart failure produce inadequate renal blood flow; this insufficiency of renal blood flow stimulates the production of salt and water-retaining hormones. This theory, called *forward* heart failure, implies that part of the problem of congestive failure develops independently of back pressure. It is very likely that both backward and forward heart failure co-exist and that the various clinical findings are a combination of both causes.

The Clinical Spectrum of Right Heart Failure

The signs and symptoms of *right heart failure* can be related fundamentally to the retention of water and sodium within the body. The end result of this fluid entrapment is an overloading of the venous system which produces the following clinical findings:

Peripheral edema

As a result of increased venous pressure (and the production of salt and water retaining hormones) fluid is forced through the capillary walls into the subcutaneous tissues of the body; this fluid collects primarily in the dependent areas of the body. Thus, in patients who are ambulatory, the feet and legs are the usual sites of peripheral edema; while among patients with acute myocardial infarction, who are bedfast, peripheral edema is most prominent over the sacral area and back (which are the dependent areas at bed rest). Rarely, peripheral edema is massive and is found throughout the entire body; this state is described as anasarca.

The presence of peripheral edema accounts for the weight gain noted among patients with right heart failure.

Ascites and pleural effusion

Edema fluid may also accumulate in the abdominal and pleural cavities through the same mechanisms described above. These effusions are much less common than peripheral edema. Pleural effusions are usually associated with advanced heart failure.

Peripheral vein distension

Elevated venous pressure in the superior vena cava typically creates distention of the neck veins. If these veins remain distended when the patient is placed in a semi-upright (45 degree angle) position it is quite likely that right heart failure is present. The nurse should observe the neck veins while feeding or bathing the patient to detect this simple, but important, diagnostic clue.

Enlarged liver

The back pressure of blood within the inferior vena cava results in venous engorgement of the liver so that the organ enlarges, becomes tender, and can be palpated on physical examination. Many patients with right sided failure describe considerable discomfort in the right upper quadrant of the abdomen from this cause. Anorexia and nausea which are common with heart failure are often the result of hepatic engorgement.

Evidence of left ventricular failure

Patients with acute myocardial infarction who develop right heart failure also can be anticipated to show signs and symptoms of *left* heart failure. (i.e., dyspnea, basal rates, and/or gallop rhythm). This interrelationship has been considered previously.

The Treatment of Right Heart Failure

Because right heart failure is characterized by the retention of water and salt, the basic aim of treatment is to correct these disturbances, while at the same time improving the myocardial performance. This is accomplished in the following ways:

Restriction of sodium intake

It is customary to limit the sodium intake to 1,000 milligrams per day (low sodium diet). The degree and duration of sodium restriction varies with the severity of failure. Even though signs of failure may not be evident, many physicians prefer to limit salt intake on a prophylactic basis for all patients during the acute phase of myocardial infarction.

Diuretic therapy

Diuretic agents are used to promote the excretion of water and salt through the kidneys as a means of combating the fluid overload associated with right heart failure. Most of these drugs act in a similar manner: they block the normal re-absorption of sodium and water in the tubules of the kidney. By inhibiting the customary return of these substances to the body, the urinary output of sodium and water is greatly increased. The effectiveness of their action can be assessed by daily measurement of the patient's body weight along with careful recordings of fluid input and urinary output.

While diuretics are usually successful in their purpose, they have the undesirable effect of causing a depletion of potassium and chloride. These latter ions are also excreted in the urine when tubular reabsorption is blocked. The loss of potassium through this drug-induced mechanism is of particular concern among patients with acute myocardial infarction because low serum potassium levels (hypokalemia) can increase myocardial excitability and cause serious ventricular arrhythmias. That hypokalemia may exist can be ascertained by certain electrocardiographic changes and by determination of blood potassium levels. When potassium depletion is marked, many patients develop lassitude, anorexia, mental confusion and decreased urinary output. Replacement of potassium (either by intravenous infusion or orally) is necessary if depletion occurs.

Digitalis

Digitalis is the cornerstone of the treatment program for heart failure. The major physiologic action of digitalis is to increase the strength of myocardial contraction; ventricular emptying is enhanced in this manner. For many years, it was assumed that digitalis was contra-indicated in the presence of acute myocardial infarction because of its potential to increase myocardial irritability and thus cause dangerous arrhythmias. It now appears as if this particular threat is less formidable than had been supposed and that digitalis can be used (although not indiscriminately) to treat heart failure associated with myocardial infarction. Unfortunately, there is only a narrow zone between effectiveness of the drug and toxicity. Overdosage of digitalis (i.e., digitalis toxicity) is manifested by certain electrocardiographic changes (as noted in the section on arrhythmias) as well as by extra-cardiac symptoms, including nausea, anorexia and vomiting. In acute myocardial infarction, where right heart failure is secondary to left heart failure, digitalis is most often employed prior to the appearance of right heart failure.

THE NURSING ROLE IN ACUTE HEART FAILURE

There are two fundamental aspects of the nursing role in the management of patients with heart failure:

1) the detection of early heart failure
2) the treatment program

The Detection of Early Heart Failure

Based on the concept that the earlier acute heart failure is treated the better will be the result, it can be appreciated why the nursing role assumes such great importance in the total management of patients with acute infarction. Because the nurse is in constant attendance (unlike the physician), and has the opportunity of following the patient's clinical course uninterruptedly, the detection of early signs of heart failure has become a fundamental part of coronary care nursing.

Successful detection of early heart failure is based on *planned, careful observation* by the nurse.

The nursing assessment should include the following observations, all of which may suggest that the left ventricle is failing:

1) **Respiration**

   Observe the rate and quality of the respiratory effort. Is the patient dyspneic? Is he more comfortable propped-up in bed? Does he cough? Is the rate of respiration changing?

2) **Pulse rate**

   Record the pulse rate regularly. Compare the rate deliberately with previous recordings. An increase in pulse rate, particularly over 100 per minute, is cause for suspicion that left heart failure exists. (This possibility becomes more likely when an obvious cause for tachycardia, e.g., temperature elevation, is not apparent).

3) **Neck vein distension**

   Observe the neck veins to see if they are distended with the head of the bed raised to a 45 degree angle. (Neck vein distension may normally be present in the recumbent position. This sign suggests failure only if the distension persists while the head and trunk are elevated).

4) **Anxiety and insomnia**

   Assess the probable basis of restlessness, anxiety, or disturbed sleep pattern. All of these symptoms may often be subtle warnings of early left ventricular failure. The indiscriminate use of sedation for these complaints without consideration of the underlying mechanism is a poor practice and may delay the early diagnosis of heart failure.

5) **Physical examination by nurses***

Examine the patient in a systematic way to detect the presence of rales and a gallop rhythm. In addition, liver tenderness and dependent edema should be sought.

If the nurse detects signs or symptoms of early heart failure, she should:

1) notify the physician of these findings promptly.

2) observe the patient carefully for progression of heart failure.

3) institute the treatment program as ordered by the physician.

The Treatment Program

Unlike the nursing role in the detection of early heart failure which centered about thoughtful observation, the nurse's responsibility with advanced heart failure is concerned not only with recognition of the problem but also with the initiation of a planned treatment program.

The Nursing Role in the Treatment of Pulmonary Edema

1) Recognize the emergency and call the physician immediately. When acute pulmonary edema develops the clinical picture is so characteristic that the nurse will usually identify this complication at once.

2) Administer oxygen by means of a tight-fitting face mask. The flow rate should be adjusted to 8-10 liters per minute.

3) Raise the head of the bed so the patient is in a semi-Fowler's or a full sitting position. This change in posture usually facilitates breathing and is particularly helpful with paroxysmal nocturnal dyspnea.

---

* The concept of nurses performing physical examination for diagnostic reasons, while perhaps removed from traditional nursing duties, has gained wide and enthusiastic acceptance. It is quite clear that repeated physical examination by nurses greatly enhances the diagnosis of heart failure in its early stages and represents an important improvement in the total care of patients with acute myocardial infarction. It seems likely that this practice will become as commonplace as the now accepted role of the nurse in the detection of arrhythmias.

4) Prepare and administer drug therapy as ordered by the physician (or in accordance with standing orders of the coronary care unit*). The customary treatment will usually include morphine, a rapid acting diuretic agent, and intravenously administered digitalis.

5) Apply rotating tourniquets if the previous procedures have not been successful.

6) Observe the monitor for the development of arrhythmias. Decreases in tissue oxygen levels and electrolyte disturbances induced by the failing circulation commonly precipitate serious arrhythmias during this period.

Other Nursing Responsibilities in the Treatment Program

There are several other nursing duties attendant to the treatment program including the following:

Measurement of urinary output and fluid intake

Effective treatment for acute heart failure is usually followed by an increase in urinary output. Careful measurement of the urinary volume is therefore an important means of assesing therapy. Because it is customary to restrict oral and intravenous fluids during and immediately after acute heart failure, the fluid intake must also be calculated with care.

Dietary restriction

As noted, restriction of sodium intake is a common practice during the acute phase of myocardial infarction. Many patients find sodium restricted diets unpalatable and the nurse should make every effort to explain the need for dietary control to the patient.

Side effects of drug therapy

Both digitalis and diuretic agents, the most commonly used drugs in treating acute heart failure, may produce undesirable effects. Digitalis, when administered in excessive amounts (digitalis toxicity) may lead to serious arrhythmias (as explained in the next chapters) and careful arrhythmic detection by the nurse is essential. The use of diuretic agents may result in hypokalemia which also predisposes to arrhythmias.

The nurse should be cognizant of these problems and recognize that many arrhythmias represent side effects of therapy.

---

* Because most hospitals do not have house officers, or physicians in full time attendance, it has become rather common for the medical staff to adopt a standard treatment program for emergency situations which the nurse may initiate if a physician is not immediately available.

CARDIOGENIC SHOCK

At the present time the most serious complication of acute myocardial infarction is cardiogenic shock; probably 80% or more of patients who develop the combination of clinical findings comprising cardiogenic shock, can be expected to die.

Although the precise cause of cardiogenic shock is still unknown, its effect is clear: an insufficiency of blood and oxygen to vital organs (inadequate perfusion) and death. This profound decrease in effective blood flow results from progressive inability of the left ventricle to effectively pump blood throughout the body. In other words, cardiogenic shock implies that left ventricular function is so decreased that tissue perfusion to the brain and other organs is inadequate to sustain life. Just why the ventricle fails in its role among certain patients with myocardial infarction is not known but two mechanisms are suspected: either the left ventricular wall has been so badly damaged by the infarction itself that it can no longer generate enough force to propel blood, or that ischemia of the myocardium creates certain derangements of muscle metabolism which inhibit effective contraction. Because this fundamental question remains unanswered currently, a specific treatment program for cardiogenic shock is not available.

Despite the lack of knowledge concerning etiology, substantial information is available about the hemodynamic consequences of cardiogenic shock. The basic hemodynamic effect is a *marked reduction in cardiac output.* Specifically, the left ventricle ejects a grossly reduced volume of blood with each contraction (decreased stroke volume) and the total amount of blood pumped per minute (i.e., the cardiac output) is reduced accordingly. In addition, the arterial blood pressure falls so that the vital organs fail to receive sufficient blood and oxygen (inadequate perfusion) to maintain cellular metabolism.

It has been supposed that the body compensates for this circulatory failure by constricting the smaller arterioles throughout the body in an attempt to confine the circulating blood volume to a smaller area and thus maintain perfusion to the vital organs. While this response of generalized vasoconstriction is undoubtedly active in shock due to blood loss, there is considerable uncertainty about the part this mechanism plays in cardiogenic shock. Believing that such vasoconstriction may be inadequate, physicians have used vasopressor drugs, hoping to increase the blood pressure and the blood flow through this means.

Unless adequate perfusion can be restored cellular death occurs. Once the vital organs are destroyed in this manner treatment is to no avail, and death must be anticipated; this state is called *irreversible shock.* The exact dividing line between irreversible and reversible shock is unknown but it appears that reversibility is related to the duration of the perfusion deficit. It is believed that certain enzyme systems concerned with tissue oxidation are irreparably damaged during cardiogenic shock and that death occurs from this cause. The occasional effectiveness of large doses of hydrocortisone in the treatment of some forms of shock suggests that adrenal gland failure may also contribute to the irreversibility of shock; however, this premise has not been proven. The end stage of cardiogenic shock is a generalized vasodilation (circulatory collapse), while the immediate cause of death is usually ventricular standstill. These agonal events are categorized as *power failure.*

The Clinical Picture Of Cardiogenic Shock

Most of the clinical findings of cardiogenic shock can be explained on the basis of reduced cardiac output and the resultant decrease in tissue perfusion. The typical picture of this profound circulatory failure includes the following signs which collectively define cardiogenic shock:

Mental Changes

One of the earliest signs of cardiogenic shock often is mental apathy and lassitude. The patient seems disinterested in his surroundings and frequently stares into space. Confusion, agitation and restlessness are other common findings. All of these mental changes reflect ineffective perfusion of the brain. As the shock state progresses, coma may develop.

Oliguria

As a result of decreased renal blood flow, the kidneys fail to function effectively and the urinary volume decreases markedly. With adequate perfusion the kidneys should excrete at least 1cc of urine per minute (or 60 cc per hour). During shock the urinary volume is diminished below this level (oliguria) or may cease entirely. This latter condition (anuria) is an ominous sign and often signals irreversible shock.

Hypotension

A fall in blood pressure is a cardinal sign of cardiogenic shock; the systolic blood pressure is usually less than 80 mm. Hg. However, it should be clearly understood that hypotension, by itself, without other accompanying signs of decreased perfusion (i.e., mental changes and oliguria) should not be construed as cardiogenic shock. For example, if a patient has a blood pressure of 80/50 but the pulse rate is not rapid, the urinary output is normal, and there is no suggestion of mental confusion; it would be unwise to categorize the problem as cardiogenic shock. A more reasonable diagnosis would be simple hypotension, a common sequela of myocardial infarction and of much less significance than shock.

As cardiogenic shock develops, the systolic blood pressure generally falls *before* the diastolic pressure so that a reading of 70/60 is not unusual in this circumstance. The numerical difference between the systolic and diastolic pressures is called the *pulse pressure* (e.g., 120/80 = pulse pressure of 40 mm. Hg.). Since reduction of the pulse pressure is an early manifestation of cardiogenic shock, careful recording of the blood pressure readings is important to detect this (sometimes insidious) change. In advanced stages of cardiogenic shock the diastolic pressure also falls and often the blood pressure is unobtainable. (It should be realized that *indirect* blood pressure measurement with the standard cuff-stethoscope technique may give spuriously low readings on certain occasions. (For this reason, many coronary care units resort to *direct* blood pressure measurement, involving the use of an indwelling arterial catheter, when standard indirect readings are not obtainable).

Cold, moist skin

Because of the marked peripheral vasoconstriction which usually accompanies shock there is a marked reduction of blood flow to the skin. Consequently, the skin becomes pale and cold. Concomitant with the vasoconstrictive response the sympathetic nervous system is stimulated; profuse sweating results. This combination of vasoconstriction and sympathetic stimulation produces the classical pale, cold, clammy skin of cardiogenic shock.

In summary, patients with cardiogenic shock can be expected to have signs of decreased perfusion involving *multiple* systems. It is the *combination* of these signs that permits the diagnosis of cardiogenic shock. One isolated finding (e.g., cold moist skin or decreased urinary output) should not be construed as cardiogenic shock.

In addition to the four classical signs of cardiogenic shock just described, these other findings usually are present:

Acute Heart Failure

When the cardiac output falls during cardiogenic shock the effective blood flow to the myocardium itself is grossly reduced. This perfusion deficit further embarrasses existing ischemia (from the infarction) and leads to acute heart failure. Thus, patients with cardiogenic shock almost always show evidence or rales, a gallop rhythm, distended neck veins, and have dyspnea.

Metabolic Acidosis

Adequate oxygenation is essential for normal cellular metabolism and function. In cardiogenic shock the supply of oxygen to the tissues is drastically reduced. Attempting to preserve cellular function and life the body employs a temporary alternate metabolic pathway which does not demand oxygen; this is called *anaerobic* metabolism in contrast to the normal *aerobic* pathway which uses oxygen. The end product of aerobic metabolism is *carbonic acid* which is excreted as carbon dioxide by the lungs while the end product of anaerobic metabolism is *lactic acid*. Unlike carbon dioxide which is readily removed from the body, lactic acid cannot be excreted by the lungs or kidneys and accumulates in the blood. This retention of lactic acid results in *acidosis*. Lethal arrhythmias, which are refractory to treatment, are common in the presence of such acidosis and cause death. Furthermore, unless lactic acidosis is corrected promptly cells cannot survive.

The Treatment of Cardiogenic Shock

Since the underlying cause of cardiogenic shock is still unknown, it is understandable why a specific treatment program for cardiogenic shock is not yet available. There is a wide diversity of opinion regarding the most effective method for combating cardiogenic shock. It is fair to say that no single approach to the problem has been successful to date; at least 70 to 80% of all patients who develop cardiogenic shock die.

At the present time the major hope for saving the lives of patients with cardiogenic shock involves a program aimed at *early detection* (long before the point of irreversibility) along with a *rational plan of therapy* designed to correct the hemodynamic disturbances.

Early detection of cardiogenic shock can only be accomplished by repeated, planned observation of the patient's clinical state. This assessment is an important nursing responsibility.

The treatment program is based on one fundamental aim: to improve left ventricular pumping function as a means of restoring adequate tissue perfusion. To accomplish this goal a variety of methods are employed including the following:

The Use of Ionotropic Agents to Improve the Strength of Myocardial Contraction.

Since the underlying defect in cardiogenic shock appears to be a reduction in cardiac output resulting from a decrease in left ventricular pumping function, it would seem logical to combat the problem by the use of drugs whose action is to increase the strength of myocardial contraction (inotropic drugs). Many believe that the use of inotropic agents should be the primary and initial method of therapy. The two most effective agents for this purpose are digitalis preparations and isoproterenal (Isuprel); the latter drug being the most potent of all inotropic agents now available.

The actual effectiveness of this approach has not been specifically proven to date. Some physicians suspect that inotropic drugs are self-limiting in effectiveness because the myocardium during cardiogenic shock is too damaged to respond to the inotropic effect.

The use of vasopressor agents to sustain the blood pressure

There is considerable debate currently about the value of vasopressor drugs in the treatment of cardiogenic shock. Some physicians feel that vasopressors (e.g., Levophed, Aramine, Wyamine, etc.) are of little importance in this situation since the peripheral vessels are probably fully constricted (as part of the body's own defense mechanism against shock) and that the use of these vasoconstrictors is not justified (particularly since these drugs may induce lethal arrhythmias). Others are convinced that vasopressors are distinctly beneficial and that they do raise the blood pressure to levels which permit adequate perfusion to the heart and brain irrespective of the degree of natural reflex vasoconstriction that may exist.

The use of sodium bicarbonate to combat lactic acidosis

It is essential that lactic acidosis be controlled if life is to be preserved. This control is accomplished by large amounts of sodium bicarbonate given intravenously.

The use of oxygen

As a means of improving tissue perfusion the administration of oxygen is considered valuable. Many believe that unless oxygen is delivered by positive pressure or other types of mechanical assistance its usefulness is reduced.

The use of mechanical means to assist the left ventricle

Assuming that cardiogenic shock is the result of extensive structural damage to the left ventricle, which any drug therapy would be unable to combat, many clinicians have concluded that the most effective means of treating cardiogenic shock is by *mechanically* assisting the failing circulation. Several types of mechanical assistance have been proposed and attempted but at the present time none of these has proven effective enough to be adopted for general use. The extent of the current research effort in this direction, however, suggests that useful equipment for this purpose will be developed in the near future.

The use of other therapeutic approaches

Many other methods of treatment have been suggested to reduce the awesome mortality from cardiogenic shock. Among these are the use of hypothermia (to reduce the metabolic demands of tissues); large amounts of intravenous steroids; plasma expanders (e.g., Dextran); and hyperbaric oxygen. While these techniques have merit conceptually, there has been no secure evidence to indicate that any of the approaches have a high degree of success; all of these methods must be considered experimental at this time.

THE NURSING ROLE IN CARDIOGENIC SHOCK

1. **The early detection of cardiogenic shock**

   Recognizing that the results of any therapy are practically hopeless once cardiogenic shock is far advanced it becomes obvious that early detection and treatment are essential if life is to be saved. The nursing role in this regard is of vital importance.

   By repeated, planned observation at the bedside, the nurse can frequently detect changes in the patient's clinical status which suggest that cardiogenic shock is developing. Specific attention should be given to the following signs:

   a) a decrease in systolic blood pressure with a narrowing of the pulse pressure.

   b) cold, moist skin

   c) a decrease in the urinary volume

   d) lethargy, anxiety, or mental confusion

2. **The treatment program**

When signs of cardiogenic shock are present, the nurse should proceed as follows:

   a) notify the physician at once.

   b) start an intravenous infusion of 5% glucose in water.

   c) administer oxygen by means of a tight fitting plastic face mask; the flow rate should be 8 - 10 liters per minute.

   d) insert an indwelling catheter into the urinary bladder and measure and record the urinary volume every 20 minutes.

   e) measure the blood pressure with great care at regular intervals. By comparing these serial readings, a continuous fall in the blood pressure can be distinguished from a stabilized level.

   f) observe the monitor repeatedly for the development of serious arrhythmias, since this latter complication is common among patients with cardiogenic shock. The defibrillator should be at the bedside.

   g) place the patient in a semi-upright position. Avoid the Trendelenburg position (used in hemorrhagic shock) as it is disadvantageous in cardiogenic shock.

   h) start the treatment program ordered by the physician.

The following basic drugs should be available:

   - Isoproterenol (Isuprel)
   - Rapid acting intravenous digitalis (ouabain, Cedilanid, etc.)
   - Sodium bicarbonate (preferably prepared 5% solutions containing about 300 millequivalents in 500 cc. bottles).
   - Vasopressor agents (Levophed, Aramine, Wyamine, etc.)
   - Rapid acting diuretics (Lasix, Edecrin)

3. **Assessment of treatment program**

In order to evaluate the effectiveness of treatment and the need for changes in the regimen, it is essential that certain physiological measurements must be made repeatedly by the nurse-physician team. The specific determinants used for these purposes will vary at different hospitals but the following measurements can be considered standard in most coronary care units: blood pressure, pulse rate, central venous pressure, blood pH and oxygen levels, and urinary output. In addition, at large hospitals more sophisticated methods including direct blood pressure measurement (utilizing indwelling arterial catheters) and determinations of cardiac output may also be used.*

THROMBOEMBOLISM

There is an unusual tendency and a high incidence of intravascular clotting among patients with acute myocardial infarction; the exact reason for this is uncertain. It may be that clots (thrombi) develop primarily as a result of the venous stasis that accompanies prolonged bed rest and muscular inactivity. However, there is some suspicion that this propensity for clotting may be inherent in patients with coronary heart disease and that there are specific factors in the blood which promote abnormal coagulation. (Those favoring the latter concept suspect that the original clot within the coronary artery may result from this same defect). There are several studies in progress attempting to answer this important question.

Most thrombi arise in either the deep veins of the legs (peripheral thrombi) or directly within the chambers of the heart (mural thrombi). The thrombi break loose from these sites, perhaps when the venous pressure is suddenly increased, and migrate as *emboli*. Depending on where they eventually lodge, emboli are classified as pulmonary, cerebral or peripheral.

Pulmonary Embolism

Unlike the cerebral or peripheral types, pulmonary emboli almost always originate in the *deep veins of the legs*. The clots pass through the right atrium, the right ventricle and finally occlude the pulmorary artery or its branches. There is little chance of *mural* thrombi causing pulmonary embolism since these latter clots are confined almost exclusively to the *left* heart and consequently remain in the systemic rather than the pulmonary circulation. In this sense, pulmonary emboli are not a direct effect of myocardial infarction but develop from secondary factors.

The true incidence of pulmonary embolism in acute myocardial infarction is difficult to evaluate since it is quite clear that the largest percentage of these episodes are not recognized before death. It would appear that occlusion of small branches of the pulmonary arteries may not produce distinct symptoms or physical findings. Postmortem studies have shown that pulmonary emboli occur in probably 25% or more of all

---

* The techniques of measuring central venous pressure and direct arterial pressure are not considered here. These methods, and the related nursing role are described in detail in "Concepts and Practices of Intensive Care for Nurse Specialists," Meltzer, Abdellah, Kitchell, The Charles Press, Inc. Philadelphia 1969.

patients with acute myocardial infarction; however, only a small percentage of these emboli are a direct cause of death. It is estimated that no more than 2%-4% of all deaths from myocardial infarction can be attributed to this particular complication. When pulmonary embolism is death-producing, the event is often sudden and follows obstruction of the main pulmonary artery.

Clinical picture of pulmonary embolism

With a large or massive pulmonary embolus the patient may describe *sudden* chest pain, on either the left or right side, which is increased by inspiration. The pain may be misinterpreted as due to additional myocardial ischemia. Dyspnea, cyanosis and cough (sometimes hemoptysis) then develop. The blood pressure generally drops and shock may follow shortly. In some instances death may occur within minutes after the onset, but the patient may survive for longer periods during which time restlessness, confusion, convulsions and air hunger may be observed. Recovery is unusual under these circumstances.

As noted in previous paragraphs, the *majority* of patients with pulmonary emboli do not show the above picture and clinical features may be non-existent or non-specific at best.

Physical and radiographic examination of the chest can sometimes confirm the diagnosis of pulmonary embolism. The lung areas deprived of blood undergo necrosis and consolidate (pulmonary infarction). This end stage may be detectable by routine chest x-ray or radioactive scanning of the lungs depending on the extent of involvement. The electrocardiogram is sometimes of help in establishing the diagnosis of pulmonary embolism because a distinctive strain pattern of the right ventricle, which develops from pumping against the great resistance created by the embolus, can be identified.

The onset of pulmonary embolism is by no means constant or predictable but its sudden occurrence after the patient strains at defecation or first gets out of bed after prolonged inactivity is common enough to deserve special attention.

Cerebral Embolism

Mural thrombi from the injured left ventricle reach the cerebral arteries and occlude these vessels producing cerebral infarction. The site of obstruction determines the clinical course and eventual outcome. This event may occur shortly after the original coronary thrombosis so that it is not uncommon for patients to be admitted with typical findings of a cerebrovascular accident (stroke) when the underlying problem is actually an acute myocardial infarction. The presence of hemiplegia, aphasia and confusion obscures the symptoms of a myocardial infarction and for this reason it is good practice to routinely take an electrocardiogram on all patients with sudden cerebrovascular disease.

Clinical picture of cerebral embolism

Most cerebral emboli do *not* cause sudden death; the usual picture is that of a stroke. The combination of an acute myocardial infarction and a cerebrovascular accident is ominous and the prognosis is extremely poor.

Peripheral Embolism

When a mural thrombus leaves the left ventricle and obstructs a *peripheral* artery, the occlusion is usually found where the artery bifurcates. The most common sites of peripheral embolization are in the femoral and iliac arteries although any artery may be involved.

Clinical picture of peripheral embolism

The picture of sudden peripheral vessel occlusion is quite distinctive and will seldom go unrecognized. There is acute pain in the involved extremity associated with coldness, pallor and loss of pulsations. Gangrene develops eventually if collateral circulation is insufficient or if the embolus is not surgically removed.

Treatment of Embolism

The best treatment is *prevention* of thrombus formation. Such prevention is the major purpose of anticoagulant therapy and there is substantial evidence in behalf of this approach. While some physicians believe that the benefit from this therapy actually does not exceed the anticipated risk associated with its use (i.e., uncontrolled bleeding), a dispassionate analysis of available data allows the conclusion that the incidence of embolism is *definitely reduced* among patients receiving anticoagulants. On the other hand, anticoagulant therapy must not be viewed as a panacea; these drugs cannot be expected to prevent deaths from shock, congestive heart failure or arrhythmias.

The frequency of thrombus formation may also be reduced by good nursing care whereby venous stasis is minimized by periodic motion of the extremities and frequent change of body position.

Once embolism has occurred in the lungs or the brain there is little that can be done in most instances. Peripheral emboli and also pulmonary emboli can be approached surgically but the operative risk is high in patients with acute myocardial infarction.

NURSING ROLE IN EMBOLISM

The responsibilities of the nurse in the treatment program are as follows:

1) Routinely and periodically change the patient's position in bed to avoid pooling of venous blood. Gently move the patient's arms and legs several times each day. Have the patient avoid straining at defection and provide stool softeners or laxatives when needed.

2) Carefully examine the patient's body during routine nursing care when anticoagulant drugs are being administered to note any evidence of abnormal bleeding (ecchymosis) into the skin. Examine urine and stools carefully for the same reason. Keep an accurate graph of prothrombin levels or clotting times for the physician's use.

3) If a patient suddenly develops chest pain, cough, or hemoptysis, the possibility of pulmonary embolization should be suspected; oxygen should be administered immediately and the physician notified. It is essential to rule out the possibility that sudden death attributed to massive pulmonary embolus is not, in fact, due to a *reversible* cause, such as ventricular fibrillation.

4) Because survival after peripheral embolism is directly related to the interval between the actual obstruction of the artery and the time blood flow is surgically re-established, the nursing responsibility in detecting this complication at its onset is of paramount importance. Any delay can increase the likelihood of irreversible damage.

VENTRICULAR RUPTURE

Rupture of the ventricle is the least common of the major complications of acute myocardial infarction. Although statistics vary, this catastrophe probably accounts for less than 5% of all deaths from acute infarction.

When the infarction is extensive, or healing is delayed for some reason, the involved area of the left ventricle may weaken, soften, and perforate suddenly. This perforation may occur in either the outer wall of the ventricle, or in the interventricular septum; the former site is much more common.

After rupture of the free ventricular wall blood rushes through the rent and fills the surrounding pericardial sac. This extravasation of blood within the closed pericardium produces a compression of the heart (cardiac tamponade) and as a result ventricular filling is markedly diminished. Death usually occurs within minutes but survival for an hour is possible.

Although the exact cause of ventricular rupture is still uncertain, it had been suspected for many years that physical activity in the immediate post-infarction period was a major factor in this catastrophe. It now appears that this concept does not adequately explain the problem since many ruptures occur despite absolute bed rest. There are some data to suggest that ventricular rupture is more frequent in patients treated with anticoagulant therapy, but again, this belief is unproven. There is increasing evidence at the present time indicating that ventricular rupture is more common in women than in men (this is the only complication of acute myocardial infarction that occurs more often in females than in males). This may relate to the prevalence of hypertension in women, since sustained high blood pressure is thought to be a contributory cause for rupture. Unlike the previous impression that ventricular rupture occurred most frequently between the 6th and 10th day after infarction it is now known that this fatal event can develop any time after an infarction, including the first 24 hour period.

When the rupture involves interventricular septum rather than the free ventricular wall, death need not occur immediately but the prognosis is extremely poor.

The Clinical Picture of Ventricular Rupture

There is no distinctive clinical pattern to suggest that rupture of the ventricular wall has occurred. Most patients with this complication die suddenly and the impression is that of an arrhythmic death. The diagnosis can sometimes be suspected by an abrupt slowing of the heart rate in the absence of other arrhythmic warnings. A needle puncture of the pericardium (a pericardial tap) with the aspiration of blood may confirm the diagnosis.

When the interventricular septum perforates the diagnosis can be established by the sudden appearance of a loud, precordial murmur which did not exist previously. This finding, coupled with the abrupt development of *right* heart failure (due to the communication between the ventricles), usually identifies septal rupture.

The Treatment of Ventricular Rupture

In most instances, because of the very short time between rupture of the ventricular wall and death, the only possible therapy, namely surgical repair of the tear, can seldom be attempted.

With interventricular septal rupture where the patient survives the immediate insult, surgical intervention may be life-saving.

The Nursing Role in Ventricular Rupture

The most important nursing responsibility in ventricular rupture is to make certain that sudden death (resulting from ventricular rupture) is not actually due to a treatable and reversible cause, specifically ventricular fibrillation or standstill

CARDIAC ARRHYTHMIAS

Arrhythmias are the most common complication of acute myocardial infarction. Probably 90% of all patients with infarction develop some disturbance in the rate or rhythm of the heart beat and prior to the introduction of the system of coronary care almost half of all infarction deaths were due to this single cause.

Because of the extreme importance of arrhythmic complications the remaining chapters of this book are dedicated to the identification and treatment of each of the common arrhythmias.

CHAPTER 9

The Electrocardiographic Basis of Arrhythmias

In order to recognize various arrhythmias and understand their treatment it is essential that nurses acquire a fundamental, usable knowledge of electrocardiography. It is only with the electrocardiogram that most arrhythmias can be positively identified.*

Fundamentals of Electrocardiography

Each normal heart beat is the result of an electrical impulse that originates in a specialized area of the right atrium called the *sinoatrial (SA) node.* This island of tissue serves as a 'battery' for the heart and normally discharges an electrical force 60-100 times a minute in rhythmic fashion. Because the SA node controls the heart rate, it is designated as the *pacemaker;* however, all areas of the myocardium have the potential ability to serve in this capacity (an inherent property of cardiac tissue) but they assume this role only under abnormal circumstances.

This original impulse is transmitted through the heart in an orderly path; when it reaches the ventricular muscles, contraction occurs.

The electrical conduction from the SA node to the ventricle is shown in the following diagram:

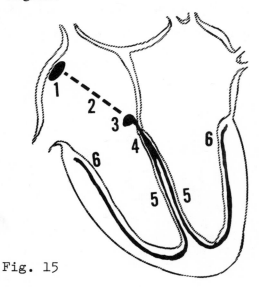

Fig. 15

a) The impulse begins in the SA node (1).

b) It spreads through the atrial muscles (2) which then contract.

c) It crosses the atrio-ventricular (AV) node (3) and passes down the Bundle of His(4).

d) Descending through the left and right bundle branches (5), the impulse finally reaches the terminal Purkinje fibers (6).

e) Ventricular contraction then occurs.

* When we conceived the system of intensive coronary care it was our impression that nurses would require a detailed course in electrocardiography, not unlike that offered to house officers. We have since found that this comprehensive program is unnecessary and that nurses can function in their intended roles with considerable less training than was given originally.

In the following discussion only the most rudimentary aspects of electrocardiography are considered. The major emphasis throughout the chapter is on the practical application of this science.

After contracting, the muscles rest and recover while the ventricles fill with blood. The next impulse normally arrives when filling is complete and ventricular contraction again occurs. The combined periods of contraction (depolarization) and recovery (repolarization) constitute the cardiac cycle.

Each fraction of the cardiac cycle is characterized by changes in the electrical activity of the heart. The original impulse from the SA node, the conduction through the heart, the contraction of muscles and the recovery period can be correlated with the flow of electrical forces at the particular instant. That this electrical activity could be detected and measured has been known since the turn of the century when Einthoven utilized a sensitive galvonometer (an *electrocardiograph*) for this purpose.

The basis of electrocardiography is straightforward: the electrical forces within the heart are transmitted outward and reach the surface of the body where they can be detected with electrodes attached to the extremities. The ebb and flow of these forces cause deflections in a galvanometer. The resulting waves are then amplified (for greater visibility) before being printed on moving graph paper. In this way a continuous "picture" of the electrical activity during the cardiac cycle is achieved. This is called an *electrocardiogram.**

Because the electrical forces from the heart extend in several directions simultaneously, it is necessary to record the flow of current in different planes, if a comprehensive view of the electrical activity is to be obtained. There are 3 major planes (called lead I, lead II, and lead III) of electrical activity which are detected with electrodes placed on the right arm, left arm, and left leg. The flow of current placed in these leads is shown in the following diagram (Fig. 16).

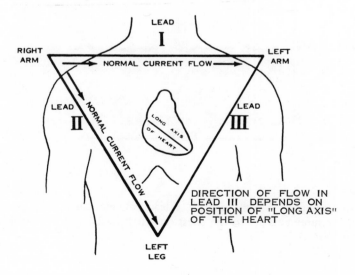

Fig. 16

---

* The instrument which detects and amplifies the electrical waves from the heart is called an *electrocardiograph*. The printed record from the *electrocardiograph* is an *electrocardiogram*.

Cardiac monitors depict a *single* lead which is the equivalent of lead II. While this is the most versatile lead for detecting a majority of arrhythmias it will by no means identify all rhythm disturbances. It is important that this limitation be recognized and when doubt exists about an arrhythmia a full 12 lead electrocardiogram must be taken.*

The electrical activity during the cardiac cycle is characterized by 5 wave deflections which are designated as P, Q, R, S, and T; the letters were arbitrarily selected and have no additional meaning.

The amplitude (or voltage) of the waves and their duration can be measured directly from the electrocardiogram.

Voltage is measured by the distance between a series of horizontal lines which are 1 millimeter apart. Each millimeter space represents one-tenth of a millivolt (the basic unit of the intensity of the electrical activity of the heart).

The *duration* of the waves is measured by the distance between a series of vertical lines, also 1 millimeter apart. The interval between vertical lines represents 0.04 seconds.

The relationship between the time and voltage is shown in the following diagram:

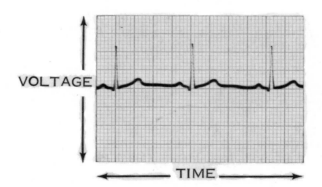

Fig. 17

* A complete electrocardiogram is composed of 12 leads which include the 3 *standard* leads (I, II, III); 6 leads concerned with measurements across the chest (called *V* leads) and 3 others which are modifications of the standard leads, (AVR, AVL, AVF).

To simplify the measurement of the wave forms every *fifth* line, both horizontally and vertically, is inscribed *boldly* producing a series of larger squares. These large squares then represent 0.5 millivolts vertically and 0.20 seconds horizontally, as shown in the following diagram:

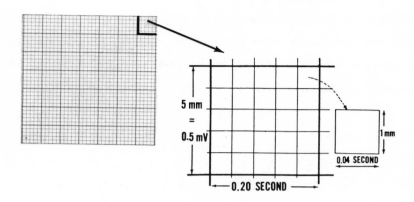

Fig. 18

The Configuration of the Normal Electrocardiogram

The electrical pattern of the cardiac cycle is seen in the accompanying

diagram.

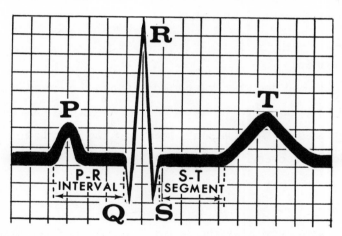

Fig. 19

The meaning and significance of the waves and time intervals follows:

P wave

This wave represents the electrical activity associated with the original impulse from the SA node and its subsequent spread through the atria.

If P waves are present, and of normal size and shape, it can be assumed that the stimulus began in the SA node; if these waves are absent or aberrant in shape, it implies that the impulse originated *outside* the SA node.

PR interval

The period from the start of the P wave to the beginning of the QRS complex is designated as the PR interval. It represents the time taken for the original impulse to pass from the SA node, through the atria and the AV node, to the ventricles.

The duration of this interval is normally less than 0.20 seconds.

If the PR interval is prolonged beyond .20 seconds, it may be assumed that a conduction delay exists in the AV node. In some instances the PR interval is unusually short (less than .10 seconds) which implies that the current reached the ventricle through a shorter-than-normal pathway (Wolff-Parkinson-White syndrome).

QRS complex

These waves represent the depolarization of the ventricular muscle and reflect the time required for the impulse to spread through the Bundle of His and its branches to complete ventricular activation. The complex consists of an initial downward deflection (Q wave), a large upward deflection (R wave) and a second downward (S wave).

The normal duration of this complex is less than 0.12 seconds. When this duration is increased it indicates that the ventricles have been stimulated in a delayed, abnormal manner (e.g., a bundle branch block).

ST segment

This interval describes the period between the completion of depolarization and the beginning of repolarization (recovery) of the ventricular muscles. The segment may be elevated or depressed if there is some injury to the muscle (e.g. acute myocardial infarction) which delays recovery.

T Wave

This wave represents the recovery phase after ventricular contraction. If repolarization is abnormal, usually because of tissue injury or ischemia, the waves may be inverted.

By analyzing these waves forms and intervals certain deductions can be made which offer enormous *indirect* information about the heart. It is important to realize that the electrocardiogram (ECG) does not depict the actual physical state of the heart or its function; it simply reflects the electrical activity of the heart. An ECG may be quite normal in the presence of heart disease unless the pathologic process actually disturbs the electrical forces. Electrocardiography has many valuable uses but its major importance is in the diagnosis of acute myocardial infarction and in the identification of abnormal rhythms.

ARRHYTHMIAS

The normal electrocardiogram consists of a repetitive series of P, Q, R, S, and T, waves, which conform to established standards for size and shape, and occur 60-100 times each minute. If these conditions prevail, the heart is in *normal sinus rhythm.* When either the rate or the contour of any of the individual waves is abnormal, the disorder is called an arrhythmia.*

Classification of Arrhythmias

There are several ways to categorize arrhythmias. Perhaps the most logical method involves classification: first, by the *site* of origin of the arrhythmia and, secondly, by the *mechanism* responsible for the disorder.

The Major *Sites* of origin of Arrhythmias Are:

SA node (sinus rhythms)

Atrial (atrial rhythms)

AV node (nodal rhythms)

Ventricles (ventricular rhythms)

The Major *Mechanisms* of Arrhythmias Are:

Tachycardia (rate greater than 100 beats per minute)

Bradycardia (rate less than 60 beats per minute)

Premature beats

Flutter

Fibrillation

Defects in conduction

On the basis of this method of classification the term *sinus tachycardia* indicates the rhythm originated normally in the sinoatrial (SA) node but that the rate is greater that 100 beats per minute (tachycardia). *Ventricular tachycardia* describes a similarly rapid rate arrhythmia which originates in the ventricles rather than in the SA node.

* In a strict sense the term arrhythmia indicates the absence of a normal rhythm and might be restricted to this one type of disturbance. In practice, however, the term arrhythmia is used collectively to describe all forms of abnormalities of the heart beat including disturbances in rate, rhythm and conduction.

Arrhythmias can also be classified in a general way (but not categorically) according to their seriousness or prognosis. This is a meaningful method for nurses caring for patients with acute myocardial infarction and the one we have found useful. Using this classification, arrhythmias may be considered as:

Minor arrhythmias. These arrhythmias are not of immediate concern and generally do not affect the circulation. They are important primarily because they frequently reflect irritability of the heart.

Major Arrhythmias. These disturbances reduce the efficiency of the heart or warn of impending danger and require prompt treatment.

Death-producing arrhythmias. These are lethal arrhythmias and immediate resuscitation is necessary to prevent death.

The most common arrhythmias are classified according to the two methods described in Table 3.

Interpretation of Arrhythmias from the Electrocardiogram

There are five basic steps which assist in the identification of arrhythmias. The electrocardiogram should be studied in an *orderly* fashion in the following manner:

Step 1. Calculate the heart rate. The two simplest methods for obtaining the rate are:

a) Count the number of R waves in a 6 inch strip of the electro-cardiographic tracing (which equals to 6 seconds). Multiply this sum by 10 to get the *rate per minute.* Since the electrocardiographic paper is marked into 3 inch intervals (at the top margin), the *approximate* heart rate can be rapidly calculated.

b) Commercially available rate calculators, which measure the distance between R waves, may be placed on the electrocardiogram and the heart rate read directly from the scale.

On the basis of heart rate alone, arrhythmias can be divided into: a) slow rate *(bradycardia),* where there are less than 60 beats per minute; b) *normal* rate, where the rate is between 60-100 per minute, and c) fast rate *(tachycardia),* where there are more than 100 beats per minute. Since several arrhythmias are characterized only by rate changes, rate calculation is essential in interpreting any electrocardiogram.

TABLE 3

CLASSIFICATION OF THE MOST COMMON CARDIAC ARRHYTHMIAS

According to Site of Origin and Mechanism:

Sino-Atrial (SA) Node Arrhythmias

Sinus Tachycardia

Sinus Bradycardia

Sinus Arrhythmia

Sinoatrial (SA) Arrest or Block

Atrial Arrhythmias

Premature Atrial Contractions (PAC)

Atrial Tachycardia

Atrial Flutter

Atrial Fibrillation

Atrial Standstill

Atrio-Ventricular (AV) Node Arrhythmias

Premature AV Nodal Contractions (PNC)

AV Nodal Tachycardia

AV Nodal Rhythm

Delayed AV Conduction

    (First Degree Heart Block)

Second Degree AV Heart Block

    (2:1 or 3:1 Block)

Complete Degree Block

    (Third Degree Block)

Ventricular Arrhythmias

Premature Ventricular Contractions (PVC)

Ventricular Tachycardia

Bundle Branch Block

Ventricular Fibrillation

Ventricular Standstill

According to Prognosis

Minor Arrhythmias

Sinus Tachycardia
Sinus Bradycardia
Sinus Arrhythmia
Premature Atrial Contractions
    (less than 6 per minute)
Premature Ventricular Contractions
    (less than 6 per minute)
Premature AV Nodal Contractions
    (less than 6 per minute)
Wandering Pacemaker

Major Arrhythmias

Sinus Bradycardia
    (rate of 50 or less)
Premature Atrial Contractions
    (more than 6 per minute)
Atrial Tachycardia
Atrial Flutter
Atrial Fibrillation
Premature Ventricular Contractions
    (more than 6 per minute)
Ventricular Tachycardia
Premature AV Nodal Contractions
    (more than 6 per minute)
AV Nodal Rhythm
Sinoatrial (SA) Arrest or Block
Delayed AV Conduction (First Degree
    Heart Block)
Second Degree AV Heart Block
Third Degree Block
    (complete heart block)
Bundle Branch Block

Death-Producing Arrhythmias

Ventricular Fibrillation
    a) primary
    b) secondary
Ventricular Standstill
    a) primary
    b) secondary

Step 2. Measure the regularity (rhythm) of the R waves. This can be done by gross observation or actual measurement of the intervals. If the R waves occur at regular intervals (with a variance of less than .12 seconds between beats) the ventricular rhythm is normal. When there are differences in R-R intervals (greater than .12 seconds), the ventricular rhythm is said to be *irregular*. This division of ventricular rhythm into regular and irregular categories assists in identifying the mechanism of many arrhythmias.

Step 3. Examine the P waves. If P waves are present and precede each QRS complex, the heart beat originates in the sinus node and a *sinus rhythm* exists. The absence of P waves or an abnormality in their position with respect to the QRS complex indicates that the impulse started outside the SA node and that an *ectopic* pacemaker is in command.

Step 4. Measure the PR interval. Normally, this interval should be between 0.10 and 0.20 seconds. Prolongation or reduction of this interval beyond these limits indicates a defect in the conduction system between the atria and the ventricles.

Step 5. Measure the duration of the QRS complex. If the width between the onset of the Q wave and the completion of the S wave is greater than 0.12 seconds (3 fine lines on the paper), an intraventricular conduction defect exists.

The Interpretation of a Specific Arrhythmia

By following these 5 steps, arrhythmias can be categorized in terms of their site or origin and their mechanism. The application of orderly analysis of an electrocardiogram is shown in the following example:

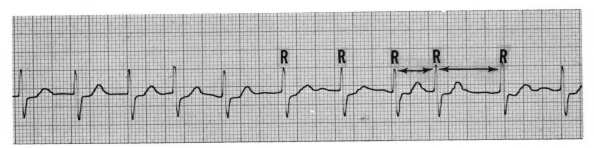

Fig. 20

1. **Rate**

   The heart rate is about 110 beats per minute, indicating that this is a fast rate arrhythmia. Note that there are 11 R waves in the 6 inch strip (11 x 10 = 110).

2. **Rhythm**

   The R-R intervals are *not* equal. We, therefore, know that this arrhythmia is characterized by an *irregular* ventricular rhythm.

3. **P waves**

   No P waves can be identified. This means that the sinus node is *not* the pacemaker and that an ectopic pacemaker exists.

4. **PR interval**

   The PR interval cannot be measured since there are no P waves.

5. **QRS complex**

   The QRS complex is .10 seconds and within normal limits (up to .12 seconds). From this fact we may surmise that the conduction through the ventricles is normal and that origin of the ectopic focus arises above the AV node (a supraventricular arrhythmia, by definition).

Analyzing this information we can reason that the abnormality originated above the AV node in the atrium, but *not* in the SA node, and is an *atrial* arrhythmia. Because the ventricular beat is *irregular*, it may be assumed that the impulse reaching the ventricles did not arrive in a rhythmic fashion. The mechanism for this particular abnormality is *fibrillation*. The electrocardiographic interpretation becomes *atrial* (site) *fibrillation* (mechanism).

ARRHYTHMIAS

The electrocardiograms shown on the following pages have been taken directly from cardiac monitors by direct write-out; they represent the patterns the nurse actually saw when she documented the arrhythmias.

It is important to realize that all of these patients had acute myocardial infarction and that many of them were also receiving drugs when the arrhythmias were recorded. As a result, most of these electrocardiograms show the latter effects in addition to the arrhythmia itself.

While 'pure' forms of the arrhythmia could have been used for these teaching purposes, we believe it is much wiser to demonstrate the arrhythmias as they are actually seen in a coronary care unit.

The methods of treatment for the individual arrhythmias described on the following pages are those we currently employ on our own service and they should not be construed as universally accepted programs. While these plans of treatment have been widely adopted, there is nevertheless a divergence of opinion in some centers about optimum treatment for several of the arrhythmias.

CHAPTER 10

Arrhythmias Originating in the Sinoatrial (SA) Node

This group of arrhythmias is caused by a relative dysfunction of the SA node.

The SA node retains its normal role as pacemaker for the heart but instead of discharging impulses at regular intervals from 60-100 times a minute, the rate extends beyond these limits (sinus tachycardia or sinus bradycardia) or the node does not discharge evenly (sinus arrhythmia).

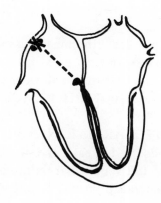

The rate and rhythm of SA node impulses is under the control of both the sympathetic and parasympathetic nervous systems. These arrhythmias result primarily from overactivity of one of these normally balanced forces. When the sympathetic system is dominant the heart rate *speeds* and when the parasympathetic system (vagus) is in control, the rate *slows*. The node itself is seldom a source of difficulty in this particular group of arrhythmias.

The conduction of the impulse after it leaves the SA node is quite normal and, therefore, the configuration of the P waves (representing atrial conduction) and the QRS complex of ventricular activation are not disturbed. The characteristic electrocardiographic pattern of these arrhythmias is simply an abnormal rate of P waves or and unevenness in their rhythm.

For the most part these arrhythmias are not serious. They most often reflect overactivity of the automatic nervous system from one of several causes. The treatment is directed at this underlying cause.

SINUS TACHYCARDIA

ETIOLOGY

The *SA node* is the pacemaker and discharges impulses at a rate of *more than 100 per minute*. This acceleration in rate usually reflects overactivity of the sympathetic nervous system resulting from either fever, anxiety, or physical activity. Sinus tachycardia often occurs through reflex mechanisms to compensate for decreased cardiac output.

CLINICAL FEATURES

1. The patient may describe palpitation and dyspnea; however, sinus tachycardia may not produce any symptoms.
2. The only pertinent physical finding is a rapid heart rate, usually 100–160 beats per minute. Sinus tachycardia must be distinguished from other rapid rate arrhythmias by ECG.
3. When sinus tachycardia returns to normal rhythm, it does so *gradually* in contrast to other tachycardias (e. g., paroxysmal atrial tachycardia) which may cease *abruptly*.

DANGER IN ACUTE MYOCARDIAL INFARCTION

1. The rapid rate tends to increase the work of the heart and its oxygen consumption. This overwork may lead to left ventricular failure or additional myocardial ischemia (angina).
2. *RISK:* The danger depends primarily on the etiology of the rapid heart rate. If sinus tachycardia is a manifestation of anxiety, fever, or physical activity, the risk is usually not significant. If sinus tachycardia is a compensatory mechanism resulting from left ventricular failure, the risk is distinctly increased and the prognosis then varies with the cardiac reserve and the duration of the tachycardia.

TREATMENT

1. The initial step in treatment is to *identify* the underlying cause of the arrhythmia rather than simply to slow the heart rate. It is particularly important to rule out the possibility that sinus tachycardia is a manifestation of early left ventricular failure.
2. Once the cause of sinus tachycardia is recognized, treatment is directed at correction of the basic problem. For example: when the rapid rate is due to temperature elevation, aspirin may be effective or, if the tachycardia is secondary to anxiety, tranquilizers or sedatives may be helpful in reducing the rate.
3. If sinus tachycardia produces ischemic pain (angina) opiates are indicated.
4. If sinus tachycardia is due to left ventricular failure, digitalis should be used.
5. Drug therapy aimed solely at reducing the heart rate, without consideration of the underlying mechanism of sinus tachycardia, is of little use.

NURSING ROLE

1. Identify the rapid rate arrhythmia as sinus tachycardia and document by a rhythm strip.
2. Examine the patient at regular intervals, always seeking possible causes for the arrhythmia, (e.g., elevated temperature, apprehension).
3. When the source of sinus tachycardia cannot be readily identified, be suspicious that left ventricular failure exists and attempt to elicit other evidence of early heart failure (e.g., orthopnea, cough, restlessness).
4. If the patient develops symptoms secondary to the arrhythmia, or if the clinical signs vary, the physician should be notified.
5. Discuss the use of sedatives, tranquilizers, aspirin, and digitalis with the physician.

SINUS TACHYCARDIA – IDENTIFYING ECG FEATURES

1. **Rate:** Usually from 100-160 beats per minute.
2. **P waves:** Normal. (If rate is very rapid, the P waves may encroach on the preceding T wave and will not be clearly identified.)
3. **QRS:** Normal.
4. **Conduction:** The entire conduction from the SA node through the ventricles is normal.
5. **Rhythm:** Regular

EXAMPLE: **Sinus Tachycardia**

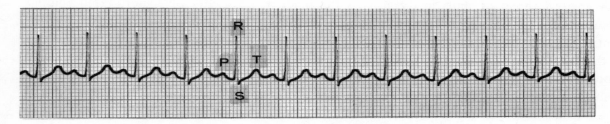

INTERPRETATION OF ECG

Rate:	About 120 per minute
P waves:	Normal.
QRS:	Normal.
Conduction:	Each P wave is followed by a QRS complex.
Rhythm:	Regular.
Comments:	Other than the rapid rate there are no other abnormalities.

EXAMPLE: **Sinus Tachycardia**

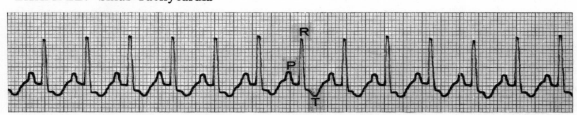

INTERPRETATION OF ECG

Rate:	About 130 per minute
P waves:	Normal.
QRS:	Normal.
Conduction:	Normal.
Rhythm:	Regular.
Comments:	The T waves are inverted reflecting myocardial ischemia.

CASE HISTORY

A 42-year-old male had been in the CCU for 2 days with a stable pulse rate ranging from 75–90 per minute. An ECG showed an acute anterior infarction with a normal sinus rhythm. While his wife was visiting, the patient became obviously upset and the monitor showed sinus tachycardia at a rate of 130 per minute. The nurse assessed the clinical condition of the patient and could find no change other than the rapid heart rate. She discussed the problem with the physician, by phone, and then administered a sedative as ordered. One hour later the pulse rate was 92.

SINUS BRADYCARDIA

ETIOLOGY

The *SA node* is the pacemaker and discharges at a rate of *less than 60 times per minute*. This slow rate is usually the result of parasympathetic (vagal) dominance of the SA node.

CLINICAL FEATURES

1. Sinus bradycardia seldom produces symptoms unless the rate is markedly decreased and reduces cardiac output.
2. The only clinical finding is a slow, regular pulse rate usually between 40—60 per minute.

DANGER IN ACUTE MYOCARDIAL INFARCTION

1. The greatest threat of sinus bradycardia is the inherent possibility of a more rapid ectopic focus assuming the pacemaker function. In this way, serious ventricular arrhythmias (e.g., ventricular tachycardia) may develop in the presence of sinus bradycardia.
2. If the heart rate is decreased enough to cause a fall in cardiac output, cerebral and coronary blood flow may become insufficient and result in syncope and/or angina.
3. Sinus bradycardia, when extreme, may be a prelude to SA node arrest and ventricular standstill; this sequence is not common.
4. *RISK:* Sinus bradycardia is associated with several *potential* dangers (described above) and for this reason, must be regarded as an important *warning* arrhythmia.

TREATMENT

1. Sinus bradycardia should be treated if any of the following circumstances exist:
   a) if premature ventricular contractions are also present.
   b) if there are signs suggesting a decreased cardiac output.
   c) whenever the rate is 50 per minute, or less.
2. Atropine, which blocks the vagal effect on the SA node, is usually effective in combating sinus bradycardia and should be the initial therapy. The drug is given intravenously in a dosage of 1.0 mg.
3. If atropine is unsuccessful, isoproterenol (Isuprel) will often increase the heart rate. The drug is administered by a slow intravenous infusion containing 1 mg isoproterenol in 500 cc glucose solution.
4. If drug therapy fails, or if its effect is short—lived, temporary transvenous pacing is often used.
5. Drugs with known bradycardic effects, such as reserpine, morphine, or propranolol, should be avoided or discontinued in the presence of sinus bradycardia.

NURSING ROLE

1. Carefully review the electrocardiogram to ascertain that the slow rate is due to sinus bradycardia rather than another cause such as heart block or a nodal rhythm. Document the arrhythmia.
2. Record the heart rate at frequent intervals for comparative purposes. This is particularly important after drug therapy is initiated.
3. Assess the patient's clinical course in a planned manner to determine if there are signs or symptoms of decreased left ventricular performance.
4. Observe the ECG pattern repeatedly for evidence of ectopic beats, particularly premature ventricular contractions. If these occur, notify the physician immediately.
5. If the heart rate falls below 50 per minute, advise the physician promptly.

SINUS BRADYCARDIA – IDENTIFYING ECG FEATURES

1. **Rate:**   Usually 40-60 per minute, but may be slower.
2. **P waves:**   Normal
3. **QRS:**   Normal.
4. **Conduction:** Each P wave is followed by a normal QRS complex.
5. **Rhythm:**   Regular.

EXAMPLE: **Sinus Bradycardia**

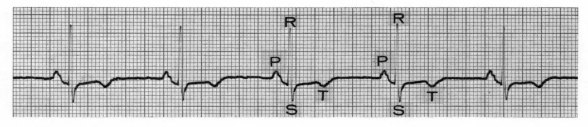

INTERPRETATION OF ECG

Rate:	About 50 beats per minute.
P waves:	Normal.
QRS:	Normal.
Conduction:	Normal conduction from SA node through the ventricles.
Rhythm:	Regular.
Comments:	The inverted T waves are not related to the arrhythmia; they result from myocardial ischemia.

EXAMPLE: **Sinus Bradycardia**

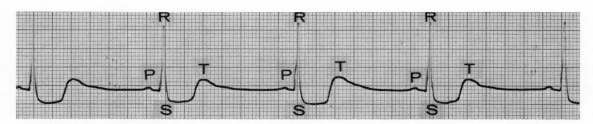

INTERPRETATION OF ECG

Rate:	42 per minute.
P waves:	Normal.
QRS:	Normal.
Conduction:	Normal; each P wave is followed by a QRS complex.
Rhythm:	Regular.
Comments:	There is deep sagging of the ST segment representing myocardial injury.

CASE HISTORY

A 52-year-old man was admitted to the unit two hours after an episode of severe chest pain. His physician had administered morphine (15 mg) at home. On arrival in the receiving ward, he was given additional morphine (8 mg) because of the persistence of chest pain. On admission to the CCU, the nurse examined the patient and found a normal blood pressure but the pulse rate was only 48 per minute. On the monitor she noted sinus bradycardia. She notified the physician and it was his impression that morphine was responsible for the bradycardia. Atropine (1.0 mg) was given intravenously and within 5 minutes the rate was 76 per minute.

SINUS ARRHYTHMIA

ETIOLOGY
The impulse originates in the *SA node* but not in a completely regular fashion. The irregularity is due to a varying influence of the autonomic nervous system on the SA node causing the rate of stimulation to *alternately* increase and decrease. In most cases, this effect is related to respiration where the rate *speeds* with inspiration and *slows* with expiration.

CLINICAL FEATURES
1. An irregular pulse is present but the patient is unaware of this minor disturbance in rhythm.
2. The diagnosis of sinus arrhythmia can only be proven by means of ECG but can be suspected clinically if the heart rate changes with deliberate breath holding.

DANGER IN ACUTE MYOCARDIAL INFARCTION
1. Sinus arrhythmia has no hemodynamic consequences, nor does it warn of more serious arrhythmias. Accordingly, it can be regarded as unimportant and non-dangerous.
2. Sinus arrhythmia should not be confused with serious causes of irregular rhythm (e.g., atrial fibrillation) and the arrhythmia is important only in this negative sense.
3. *RISK:* None.

TREATMENT
No treatment is indicated.

NURSING ROLE
Ascertain that the irregularity is sinus arrhythmia and document with ECG strip. Rule out other possible causes of irregular rhythm.

CASE HISTORY
An 82-year-old woman was admitted to the unit with typical signs of acute infarction. When taking the pulse, the nurse noted an irregular rhythm; the rate averaged 72 per minute. When the monitor was attached, she recognized that the problem was sinus arrhythmia, and recorded this on the admission sheet. This rhythm continued all during the patient's stay in the unit. No treatment was given for this minor arrhythmia.

SINUS ARRHYTHMIA — IDENTIFYING ECG FEATURES

1. **Rate:** The rate per minute is normal (60-100); however, there are variations within this period with the rate increasing momentarily during inspiration and then slowing during expiration.
2. **P waves:** Normal.
3. **QRS:** Normal.
4. **Conduction:** Each P wave is followed by QRS complex.
5. **Rhythm:** Slightly irregular due to variation in the R-R interval which varies by .12 seconds or more between the longest and shortest intervals.

EXAMPLE: **Sinus Arrhythmia**

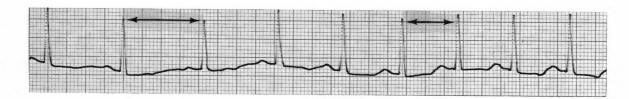

INTERPRETATION OF ECG

Rate: About 90 per minute.
P waves: Normal.
QRS: Normal.
Conduction: Normal; each P wave is followed by a QRS complex.
Rhythm: Irregular. The time varies more than .12 sec. between the longest and shortest R-R intervals.
Comments: The flat or inverted T waves are due to myocardial ischemia and are unrelated to the arrhythmia.

EXAMPLE: **Sinus Arrhythmia**

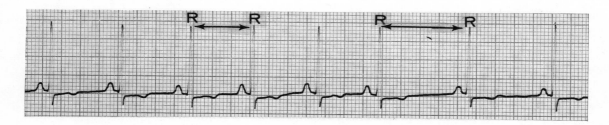

INTERPRETATION OF ECG

Rate: About 80 per minute.
P waves: Normal.
QRS: Normal.
Conduction: Normal.
Rhythm: There is a variation in R-R intervals of more than .12 seconds.
Comments: The short R-R intervals occur during inspiration. The long R-R intervals occur during expiration.

SINOATRIAL (SA) ARREST OR BLOCK

ETIOLOGY

Under certain circumstances, the SA node fails to initiate an impulse at the expected time in the cardiac cycle. In the absence of this impulse, neither the atria nor ventricles are stimulated and the entire PQRST complex drops out for one beat. This is called *sinoatrial (SA) arrest*. In some instances, the impulse is initiated normally, but is blocked *within* the node and fails to reach the atria. Again, the complete PQRST complex is absent. This condition is designated as *SA block*. Clinically, SA block and SA arrest cannot be distinguished with certainty from each other, and the terms are used interchangeably.

The usual cause of SA arrest is excessive vagal dominance of the node, but over-dosages of digitalis and quinidine must always be suspected. Ischemia of the SA node may be an underlying cause of the arrhythmia.

CLINICAL FEATURES

1. Patients may be aware of the prolonged pause reflecting the missed beat (or beats) and describe this sensation; however, most patients are unaware of the arrhythmia.
2. The only physical finding is the detection of a prolonged pause while taking the pulse or listening to the heart beat.
3. If the missed beats occur frequently or consecutively, cerebral insufficiency manifested as syncope or vertigo may develop.

DANGER IN ACUTE MYOCARDIAL INFARCTION

1. When infrequent, SA arrest is not of great importance and merely reflects vagal overactivity.
2. When related to overdosages of digitalis or quinidine, the arrhythmia assumes added significance because continuation of the drug may lead to advanced depression of SA node activity and result in atrial standstill (see page 140).
3. *RISK:* Usually not significant, but potentially serious if drug induced, or if the episodes are repetitive or prolonged.

TREATMENT

1. If the SA arrest occurs occasionally, and is secondary to excessive vagal influence, the condition is usually self-limiting and requires no treatment.
2. If periods of SA arrest are frequent or prolonged, atropine (1.0 mg intravenously) will inhibit the vagal effect on the SA node and usually permit normal initiation of the SA impulse. Isoproterenol can also be used for this purpose.
3. If SA arrest develops in patients receiving digitalis or quinidine, these drugs should be discontinued promptly.
4. Occasionally, SA arrest fails to subside spontaneously or to respond to drug therapy. In this situation, transvenous pacing is indicated.

NURSING ROLE

1. When SA arrest is noted, document the arrhythmia with a rhythm strip.
2. If SA arrest becomes frequent, or if more than two consecutive beats are missed, notify the physician promptly.
3. If SA arrest develops in patients receiving digitalis or quinidine, further dosages of these drugs should be withheld until approved by the physician.

SINOATRIAL (SA) ARREST OR BLOCK – IDENTIFYING ECG FEATURES

1. **Rate:** Usually normal but frequently in bradycardic range.
2. **P waves:** No P wave with the missed beat since the SA node either did not discharge or the impulse failed to reach the atrium.
3. **QRS:** No QRS complex is produced when the SA node impulse is absent.
4. **Conduction:** The entire PQRST complex is missing for one or more beats during sinus arrest.
5. **Rhythm:** The basic rhythm is normal except for the missing beats.

EXAMPLE: **Sinoatrial (SA) Arrest or Block**

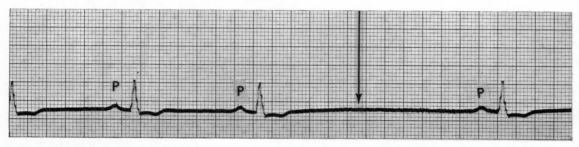

INTERPRETATION OF ECG

Rate: About 45 per minute.

P waves: The P wave anticipated after the 3rd complex is absent (see arrow).

QRS: There is no QRS complex in the absence of SA node stimulation.

Conduction: One PQRST complex is missing because of sinus arrest.

Rhythm: Sinus bradycardia with irregularity due to missed beat.

Comments: The SA node failed to discharge for one beat and then resumed its function.

EXAMPLE: **Sinoatrial (SA) Arrest or Block**

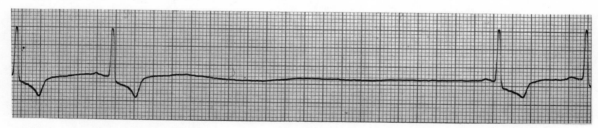

INTERPRETATION OF ECG

Rate: The underlying rate is about 60 per minute.

P waves: Following the second QRS complex, P waves do not appear during a period equivalent to three anticipated beats.

QRS: Absent when the SA node failed to discharge.

Conduction: Three entire PQRST complexes are missing (missed beats).

Rhythm: The period of SA arrest creates an irregular rhythm.

Comments: After treatment with atropine the SA block disappeared.

CASE HISTORY

A 72-year-old man was admitted with an acute posterior infarction and evidence of congestive heart failure. He was treated with digoxin, intravenously, after which oral digitalis was started. Because the heart rate remained rapid, additional digitalis was administered. On the third day, the nurse noted a slight irregularity in the rhythm of the pulse, and recognized SA arrest on the monitor. A missed beat occurred after every fifth contraction. She called the physician, and digitalis was discontinued. Episodes of sinus arrest persisted for the next 24 hours and then disappeared.

WANDERING PACEMAKER

ETIOLOGY

The *SA node* remains the basic pacemaker but at times the impulse may originate in different portions of the node, or the pacemaker may actually wander from the SA node to the AV node. This shifting of the impulse site within the SA node, or to the AV node, is usually related to vagal influences, and a wandering pacemaker is a variant of sinus arrhythmia in this respect.

CLINICAL FEATURES

A wandering pacemaker produces no symptoms or signs and can only be recognized by ECG.

DANGER IN ACUTE MYOCARDIAL INFARCTION

1. There is no particular danger from a wandering pacemaker. The arrhythmia usually reflects depression of the SA node by vagal influence.
2. *RISK:* None

TREATMENT

1. No treatment is needed in most instances.
2. If depression of the SA node permits the AV node to assume the pacemaker role increasingly, atropine can be used to block the vagal influence.
3. If a wandering pacemaker develops during digitalis therapy, the drug may be withheld temporarily to see if the arrhythmia will disappear.

NURSING ROLE

1. When a wandering pacemaker is noted on the monitor, document the arrhythmia with a rhythm strip.
2. Observe the electrocardiogram subsequently to verify that the SA node has not relinquished complete control to the AV node (nodal rhythm).

CASE HISTORY

A 54-year-old man showed evidence of a wandering pacemaker on the monitor, three days following an acute anterior infarction. Within minutes a normal sinus rhythm was again evident. During the next few hours there were several occurrences of similar episodes. The nurse noted these changes, but was not concerned about their significance since the SA node remained the dominant pacemaker throughout.

```
┌─────────────────────────────────────────────────────────────────────────────┐
│           WANDERING PACEMAKER — IDENTIFYING ECG FEATURES                      │
```

1. **Rate:**   Usually normal but may be slow (because of vagal dominance).
2. **P waves:**   As the pacemaker wanders within the SA node, or to the AV node, the shape and position of the P waves vary reflecting the different sites of origin of the impulse.
3. **QRS:**   Normal.
4. **Conduction:**   Conduction *from* the AV node to the ventricles is normal; but conduction *to* the AV node depends on the site of the impulse. Nevertheless, there is a normal QRS complex regardless of the size, shape, or position of the P waves.
5. **Rhythm:**   Normal.

EXAMPLE: **Wandering Pacemaker**

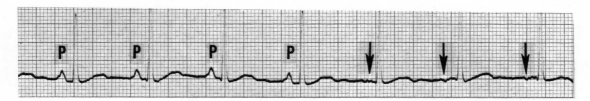

INTERPRETATION OF ECG

Rate: About 70 per minute.
P waves: The first 4 beats show normal P waves originating in the SA node. The last 3 complexes show abnormal P waves; the pacemaker has left the SA node.
QRS: Normal.
Conduction: Normal.
Rhythm: Regular.
Comments: The pacemaker wanders between the SA and AV node.

EXAMPLE: **Wandering Pacemaker**

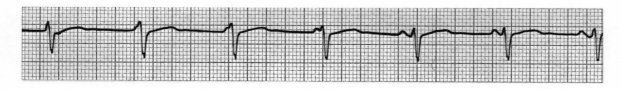

INTERPRETATION OF ECG

Rate: About 70 per minute.
P waves: There is a change in shape and position of the P waves from the first to the last complexes.
QRS: Normal.
Conduction: Normal.
Rhythm: Regular.
Comments: The pacemaker was originally in the AV node and progressively moved to the SA node.

CHAPTER 11

Arrhythmias Originating in the Atria

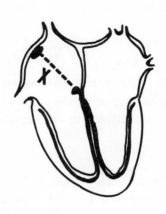

As noted previously the atria, the AV node and the ventricles all have the *potential* capacity to serve as pacemaker; but the SA node retains control because it normally discharges impulses at an inherently faster rate than the other sites. If for some reason impulses from foci in the atrial walls occur more frequently than those from the SA node, the ectopic site in the atria replaces the SA node as pacemaker. This may occur for only one beat (premature atrial contraction) or continuously (e.g., atrial fibrillation) depending on the degree and persistence of irritability of the abnormal focus.

When the impulse originates in the atria, outside the SA node, at rates of *less than 200 per minute*, the P waves are usually visible but are distorted in shape indicating that the SA node is *not* in command. With atrial rates up to 200 per minute the impulses reach the AV node and pass through to the ventricles without difficulty. Accordingly, a normal QRS complex follows each P wave.

When the atria contract *200-400 times a minute*, the AV node is unable to accept each impulse and blocks every second, third or fourth beat. The impulses that do reach the ventricles are conducted normally thereafter. For example, in atrial flutter the atrial rate is two or three times greater than the ventricular response and there are two or three P waves for each normal QRS complex.

If the atria are stimulated at extremely fast rates *(up to 1000 per minute)* the atrial muscles are no longer able to respond to each stimulus and the individual fibers, comprising the muscle, merely twitch or fibrillate. Atrial contraction ceases and P waves are no longer evident. Impulses pass the AV node in irregular fashion so that the ventricular rhythm becomes irregular as well (atrial fibrillation).

Atrial arrhythmias result primarily from irritability of the muscle walls caused by tissue damage (ischemia) or by drugs. Most atrial rhythm disturbances are dangerous and are therefore classified as major arrhythmias. Atrial arrhythmias have the ability to increase the ventricular rate and thereby decrease the effectiveness of the heart's pumping action. These arrhythmias must not be allowed to persist once they are recognized and drug therapy or precordial shock should be used to terminate them promptly.

PREMATURE ATRIAL CONTRACTIONS (PAC)

ETIOLOGY

When an ectopic focus in the atrium supersedes the *SA* pacemaker for one beat, a *premature atrial contraction* results. These ectopic beats reflect irritability of the atrial muscle. Except for these isolated premature contractions the SA node remains as the basic pacemaker.

CLINICAL FEATURES

1. Normally the patient is unaware of premature atrial contractions; however, with a stethoscope the occurrence of a beat sooner than expected may be heard.
2. Positive identification can only be made by ECG.

DANGER IN ACUTE MYOCARDIAL INFARCTION

1. By themselves PAC's have no particular significance; however, they indicate atrial irritability and may forewarn of impending serious atrial arrhythmias, e.g., paroxysmal atrial tachycardia or atrial fibrillation. When PAC's increase beyond 6 per minute, the arrhythmia assumes more importance in this regard.
2. *RISK:* No immediate danger but may herald the onset of atrial fibrillation or other atrial arrhythmias.

TREATMENT

1. If PAC's occur rarely and do not increase in frequency, treatment is usually unnecessary.
2. If the number of PAC's increase during a period of observation, it is advisable to use antiarrhythmic drugs to control these ectopic beats. Quinidine, administered orally, is probably the most effective drug in this situation.

NURSING ROLE

1. Distinguish PAC's from other causes of irregular heart rhythm and document their presence on ECG.
2. Carefully observe the frequency of these premature beats for comparative purposes and advise physician of any increase in the number of these beats.
3. Be aware that atrial fibrillation or other serious atrial arrhythmias may develop in the presence of frequent premature atrial beats.

CASE HISTORY

A 62-year-old woman had occasional premature atrial contractions during the first 24 hours after her admission. These occurred at a rate of 1-2 per minute and were duly noted by the nurse and recorded as such on each hourly ECG strip. Early in the morning of the second day, the frequency of PAC's increased to 4-5 per minute and remained at that rate. The nurse advised the physician of this change during his visit and quinidine therapy was started. Within 12 hours, the arrhythmia was no longer evident.

PREMATURE ATRIAL CONTRACTION (PAC) — IDENTIFYING ECG FEATURES

1. **Rate:**   Usually normal.
2. **P waves:**   Either abnormally shaped, or inverted, and differ from normal P wave of SA nodal origin.
3. **QRS:**   Usually normal.
4. **Conduction:** A normal QRS complex follows the abnormal P wave. There is slight delay before the next normal beat; however, this interval is usually less than the compensatory pause seen after premature *ventricular* contractions.
5. **Rhythm:**   Except for the atrial contraction which occurs prematurely, the remaining rhythm is entirely normal.

EXAMPLE: **Premature Atrial Contraction**

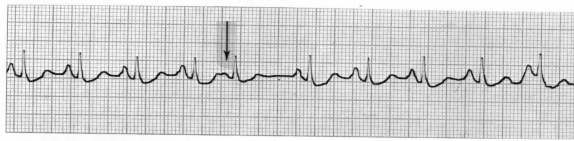

INTERPRETATION OF ECG

Rate: About 100 per minute.

P waves: The P wave of the premature beat (see arrow) is abnormally shaped and differs from the normal P waves originating in the SA node.

QRS: Normal.

Conduction: The PAC originates in the atrium but not in the AV node. The conduction is otherwise normal.

Rhythm: The premature beat and the pause that follows, create a slight irregularity in the rhythm.

Comments: Isolated premature contractions of this type are common and seldom pose a problem.

EXAMPLE: **Premature Atrial Contraction**

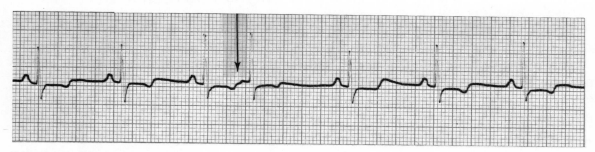

INTERPRETATION OF ECG

Rate: About 70 per minute.

P waves: Distorted with the premature beat (see arrow); the remaining P waves are normal.

QRS: Normal.

Conduction: Normal, other than site of impulse formation in the premature beat.

Rhythm: The normal rhythm is interrupted by the premature beat.

Comments: The normal QRS complex associated with a premature beat readily distinguishes the atrial origin of the impulse.

PAROXYSMAL ATRIAL TACHYCARDIA (PAT)

ETIOLOGY
An irritable focus within the atrium, but outside the SA node, becomes the pacemaker and causes the *atrium to beat 140-250 times per minute.* The ventricle is able to respond to each atrial impulse and therefore the *ventricular and atrial rates are identical.*

CLINICAL FEATURES
1. Characteristically, PAT occurs *suddenly* and without warning, but may be preceded by premature atrial contractions (occurring singly or in runs).
2. Most patients are immediately aware of the rapid heart action and frequently describe a fluttering sensation in the chest along with lightheadedness.
3. The arrhythmia may end as *abruptly* as it started even without treatment.

DANGER IN ACUTE MYOCARDIAL INFARCTION
1. The rapid heart rate tends to reduce cardiac output because the volume of blood ejected with each contraction (stroke volume) is decreased as a result of the short ventricular filling time. This decrease in cardiac output leads to left ventricular failure, particularly if the tachycardia is sustained.
2. The rapid rate increases the oxygen demand and consumption of the myocardium. This may lead to additional myocardial ischemia and the occurrence of angina. The longer PAT persists the greater the threat of further myocardial damage.
3. *RISK:* A dangerous arrhythmia in acute myocardial infarction, but not an immediate cause of death. The risk is directly proportional to the duration of PAT.

TREATMENT
1. An attempt should be made initially to terminate the arrhythmia by reflex vagal stimulation (carotid sinus massage or eyeball pressure).
2. If PAT produces angina and/or evidence of left ventricular failure and cannot be terminated by vagal stimulation, elective precordial shock should be given promptly; this latter method is predictably successful. (See Chapter 15)
3. If the rapid rate does *not* produce obvious symptoms, morphine, given intravenously, is often effective in halting the arrhythmia.
4. If PAT occurs repetitively, drug therapy can be used to prevent subsequent episodes. The choice of drugs for this purpose includes: a) rapid acting digitalis preparations (ouabain or cedilanid) given intravenously, b) quinidine, orally, c) propranolol administered either orally or intravenously.

NURSING ROLE
1. The onset of PAT will trigger the high rate alarm system of the monitor.
2. Examine the patient and verify the rapid pulse rate.
3. Document the arrhythmia with a rhythm strip.
4. Notify the physician immediately.
5. Assess the patient's clinical status, with particular reference to the presence of angina or signs of left ventricular failure. Record the blood pressure.
6. If the patient has signs or symptoms related to the arrhythmia, prepare for elective cardioversion.
7. Have appropriate drugs ready for use at the bedside.

```
PAROXYSMAL ATRIAL TACHYCARDIA (PAT) — IDENTIFYING FEATURES
```

1. **Rate:**   140-250 per minute.
2. **P waves:**   May be buried in either the QRS complex or T waves and not visible; or may be abnormally shaped.
3. **QRS:**   Usually normal but may be widened.
4. **Conduction:** A ventricular complex follows *each* P wave.
5. **Rhythm:**   Regular.

EXAMPLE: **Paroxysmal Atrial Tachycardia**

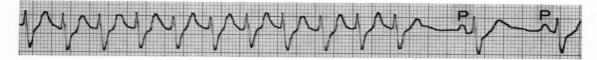

INTERPRETATION OF ECG

Rate:	About 150 per minute.
P waves:	Not visible; probably buried in the T waves.
QRS:	Essentially normal.
Conduction:	Each atrial stimulus is conducted normally causing a regular ventricular response.
Rhythm:	Regular.
Comments:	The episode of paroxysmal tachycardia stopped abruptly as noted in the last two complexes where normal sinus rhythm has returned.

EXAMPLE: **Paroxysmal Atrial Tachycardia**

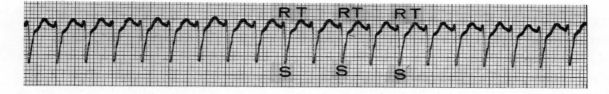

INTERPRETATION OF ECG

Rate:	200 per minute.
P waves:	Not identified.
QRS:	Essentially normal. The small R wave and deep S wave are due to the position of the skin electrodes.
Conduction:	Normal atrial and ventricular conduction.
Rhythm:	Completely regular.
Comments:	This very rapid rate arrhythmia increases the work of the heart and must be terminated promptly.

CASE HISTORY

A 55-year-old woman with an acute infarction had been in normal sinus rhythm for 48 hours since admission. At 4 P.M. the pulse rate was 82 and regular and an hourly ECG strip taken by the nurse showed a normal sinus rhythm. At 4:10 P.M. the tachycardia alarm sounded and the monitor showed a heart rate of 160. At the bedside the nurse confirmed the rapid rate. The patient complained of chest pain and was obviously frightened. The nurse ran a rhythm strip and recognized paroxysmal atrial tachycardia. She called the physician immediately and prepared for precordial shock. By the time the physician arrived, several minutes later, the arrhythmia had stopped abruptly. In reviewing the rhythm strip it was apparent that the patient had a run of PAT which lasted for less than 3 minutes.

ATRIAL FLUTTER

ETIOLOGY
The SA node is replaced as the pacemaker by an extremely irritable focus within the walls of the atrium which stimulates the atria to contract *250-400 times per minute.* The AV node *blocks* most of these atrial impulses but allows every 2nd, 3rd, or 4th impulse to reach the ventricles and cause contraction. The ventricular rate therefore varies with the degree of block in the A-V node.

CLINICAL FEATURES
1. The occurrence of symptoms depends primarily on the ventricular rate. If the ventricular response is rapid, the patient may describe palpitations, angina, or dyspnea. If the ventricular rate is normal, the patient may be unaware of the arrhythmia.
2. Atrial flutter can only be identified by means of ECG.

DANGER IN ACUTE MYOCARDIAL INFARCTION
1. When atrial flutter is associated with a rapid ventricular rate, the cardiac output may be decreased and the myocardial oxygen consumption increased (as with other rapid rate arrhythmias, e.g., PAT). This impairment predisposes to left ventricular failure and additional myocardial ischemia.
2. If the ventricular rate is not increased, left ventricular performance may not be affected significantly.
3. *RISK:* A serious arrhythmia because of the potential hemodynamic consequences.

TREATMENT
1. Atrial flutter can be predictably terminated by synchronized precordial shock; very low discharge energies (50 watt seconds or less) are required. For this reason, precordial shock should be the initial therapy, particularly when the ventricular rate is rapid.
2. Digitalis is often effective in terminating atrial flutter as well as in preventing its recurrence. A rapid-acting preparation (ouabain, cedilanid) is usually given intravenously for this purpose.
3. Other drugs, particularly quinidine or propranolol, can be used to treat atrial flutter; however, these are less desirable choices than precordial shock or digitalis in the *presence of acute myocardial infarction.*

NURSING ROLE
1. When atrial flutter develops the high rate alarm may or may not sound, depending on the *ventricular* rate.
2. Identify the arrhythmia on the monitor and document with a rhythm strip.
3. Assess the patient's clinical status. Determine if the patient has angina or dyspnea. Record the blood pressure and pulse rate.
4. Notify the physician promptly after this arrhythmia is identified.
5. If the patient complains of angina or if there is evidence of left ventricular failure, prepare for elective cardioversion. (See Chapter 15)
6. If digitalis or other drugs are used to treat atrial flutter, carefully follow the heart rate and rhythm response.

ATRIAL FLUTTER — IDENTIFYING ECG FEATURES

1. **Rate:** The ventricular rate may vary from 60-150 depending on the number of atrial impulses passing through the AV node.

2. **P waves:** There are characteristic atrial oscillations described as "saw tooth" waves which are easily identifiable. These waves (called "flutter waves") occur regularly at a rate of 250 to 400 per minute.

3. **QRS:** The QRS complex is normal.

4. **Conduction:** Only 1/2, 1/3, or 1/4 of the atrial impulses are conducted through the AV node and reach the ventricle. The resulting disparity between atrial and ventricular rates is described as atrial flutter with 2:1, 3:1, or 4:1 block. Conduction beyond the AV node is not disturbed.

5. **Rhythm:** The ventricular rhythm is most often regular. However, as a result of variations in the degree of block in the AV node from time to time, the ventricular rhythm may become somewhat irregular.

EXAMPLE: **Atrial Flutter**

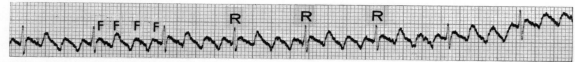

INTERPRETATION OF ECG

Rate: About 80 per minute.

P waves: There are four "F waves" between R waves (the first being buried in the T waves).

QRS: Normal.

Conduction: Every fourth "F wave" is conducted to the ventricle while 3 are blocked by the A-V node. This is designated as 4:1 block.

Rhythm: Regular.

Comments: The classical "saw tooth" appearance typifies atrial flutter.

EXAMPLE: **Atrial Flutter**

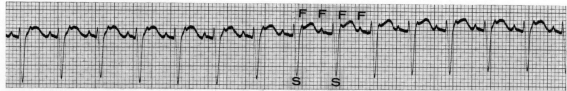

INTERPRETATION OF ECG

Rate: 150 per minute.

P waves: There are two F waves for each QRS complex; one occurs in the T wave and may not be obvious at first glance.

QRS: Normal.

Conduction: Every second atrial impulse (F wave) is blocked at the A-V node. This is called atrial flutter with 2:1 block.

Rhythm: Regular.

Comments: The F waves do not produce the typical "saw tooth" appearance here because of the lead used for arrhythmia detection.

CASE HISTORY

Six hours after his admission to the unit, a 71-year-old man developed atrial flutter. This was noted by the nurse when the high rate alarm sounded. The ventricular rate was 150 per minute. The nurse went to the bedside and noted that the patient was apprehensive. He complained of sudden shortness of breath. She immediately notified the physician and then recorded the blood pressure, pulse rate, and documented the arrhythmia. Anticipating that precordial shock would be used, in view of the circulatory impairment induced by the arrhythmia, the nurse prepared for cardioversion. This procedure was accomplished as soon as the physician arrived, and normal sinus rhythm was restored. The patient's symptoms disappeared promptly.

ATRIAL FIBRILLATION

ETIOLOGY

An ectopic focus *within the atrium* discharges impulses at a rate greater than 400 per minute. The atrial muscles cannot recover from the previous contraction before the next impulse arrives, and, as a result, these muscles do not contract uniformly. Instead, individual atrial fibers respond as they recover and the total effect is merely a twitching of the atrial wall rather than true contraction of the atrium. In this sense the atria are no more than quivering tubes connecting the great veins with the ventricles and are of no assistance in filling the ventricles.

The AV node cannot conduct the atrial impulses at this extremely rapid rate, and allows only a small percentage of these stimuli to reach the ventricular conduction system. The impulses passing the AV node do so in an irregular fashion which creates an irregular ventricular rhythm.

When the *ventricular* response (rate) is greater than 100 per minute atrial fibrillation is said to be *uncontrolled*. A ventricular rate of less than 100 is termed *controlled* atrial fibrillation.

CLINICAL FEATURES

1. Most patients are aware of the irregular heart action. Palpitations, which are frequently disturbing, are usually more prominent when the ventricular rate is uncontrolled.
2. The *irregular* heart rate and rhythm are so typical of atrial fibrillation that this clinical finding by itself is almost diagnostic of the arrhythmia.
3. A pulse deficit is usually apparent with the apical rate exceeding the peripheral pulse rate. This inequality results from variations in the volume of blood ejected with each heart beat; at times, the volume is inadequate to produce a peripheral pulse.
4. If the ventricular response is persistently *uncontrolled* evidence of a circulatory deficit manifested by angina and left ventricular failure may be anticipated.

DANGER IN ACUTE MYOCARDIAL INFARCTION

1. The major threat from this arrhythmia is reduction in the pumping efficiency of the heart (decreased cardiac output). This inefficiency results from both the rapid ventricular rate and the loss of atrial contraction. (The atrium serves as a booster pump for ventricular filling and the absence of atrial contraction can cause a 20% reduction in cardiac output). This hemodynamic deficit may lead to left ventricular failure and additional myocardial ischemia.
2. During atrial fibrillation there is a propensity for clots to form within this non-contracting chamber. Mural thrombi, with subsequent embolization, may develop on this basis.
3. *RISK:* A dangerous arrhythmia from a hemodynamic standpoint, especially when the ventricular rate is uncontrolled.

TREATMENT

1. The treatment of atrial fibrillation depends fundamentally on whether the arrhythmia is associated with circulatory insufficiency. If a patient develops left ventricular failure or angina as a consequence of atrial fibrillation, the arrhythmia should be terminated without delay by means of synchronized precordial shock.
2. If atrial fibrillation is *not* accompanied by signs of impaired circulation, then drug therapy should be attempted initially. Digitalis is the cornerstone of this program. The drug controls the rapid ventricular rate by increasing the degree of block at the AV node, but does not necessarily restore normal sinus rhythm.
3. Quinidine can be used to convert atrial fibrillation to normal sinus rhythm and while successful in many circumstances, its effect may be too slow when left ventricular failure exists.
4. If atrial fibrillation is *controlled* and of long-standing origin, (unrelated to the acute infarction) attempts to restore normal sinus rhythm may not be indicated.

ATRIAL FIBRILLATION – IDENTIFYING ECG FEATURES

1. **Rate:** Heart rate varies according to the ventricular response. It may be under 100 beats per minute (controlled atrial fibrillation) or faster (uncontrolled atrial fibrillation).

2. **P waves:** There are no true P waves, but there are rapid, small irregular waves not resembling each other called "f" (fibrillatory) waves.

3. **QRS:** The complexes are normal in shape and duration but occur *irregularly*. This irregularity is the most typical finding of atrial fibrillation.

4. **Conduction:** The conduction in the atria is bizarre. Most of the atrial impulses which bombard the AV node are blocked but those which do pass through the AV node are conducted normally thereafter. This conduction pattern is manifested by the absence of P waves and the presence of irregularly occurring, but normally shaped, QRS complexes.

5. **Rhythm:** Ventricular rhythm is totally irregular.

EXAMPLE: **Controlled Atrial Fibrillation**

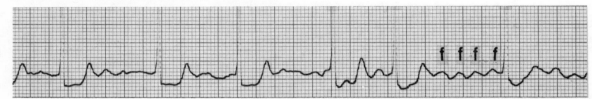

INTERPRETATION OF ECG

Rate: About 70 per minute.

P waves: No P waves are identified. Fibrillatory waves (f waves) occur irregularly.

QRS: Normal.

Conduction: Most atrial impulses are blocked at the A-V node; those that pass through are conducted normally.

Rhythm: Grossly irregular.

Comments: The irregular ventricular rhythm in conjunction with f waves is characteristic of atrial fibrillation.

NURSING ROLE

1. *If atrial fibrillation develops abruptly, or is present and uncontrolled at the time of admission:*
   a) Document the arrhythmia with rhythm strip and notify the physician.
   b) Ascertain if the arrhythmia is obviously compromising circulatory efficiency. Inquire specifically if the patient has chest pain or dyspnea.
   c) Record the pulse rate, the extent of the pulse deficit and the blood pressure.
   d) Prepare for elective cardioversion and have intravenous digitalis preparations at bedside.

2. *If atrial fibrillation is controlled or existed before the present infarction:*
   a) Observe the patient's clinical status in a planned manner at regular intervals always seeking evidence of left ventricular failure. Carefully record pulse rate, apical rate and blood pressure.
   b) Obtain serial rhythm strips at regular intervals for comparative purposes.
   c) Advise the physician of any significant increase or decrease of the ventricular rate, or if signs or symptoms develop which suggest left ventricular failure.

3. If digitalis or quinidine are used to treat atrial fibrillation observe the electrocardiogram for signs of drug overdosages. If the ventricular rate falls below 60 per minute further administration of drugs should be discussed with the physician.

4. Because of the possibility of embolization secondary to atrial fibrillation careful clinical assessment should always recognize this potential threat.

138

EXAMPLE: **Uncontrolled Atrial Fibrillation**

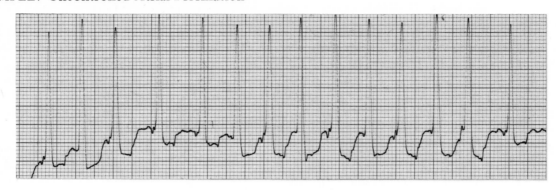

INTERPRETATION OF ECG

Rate: About 150 per minute.
P waves: P waves are not identified; the oscillations of the baseline represent "f" waves.
QRS: Normal.
Conduction: Conduction beyond the AV node is normal.
Rhythm: Irregular.
Comments: Because the ventricular rate is greater than 100 per minute, the atrial fibrillation
                  is uncontrolled.

EXAMPLE: **Atrial Fibrillation being controlled with digitalis**

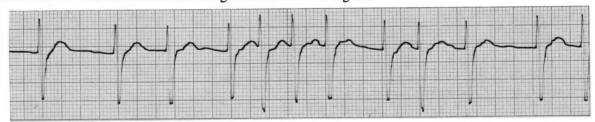

INTERPRETATION OF ECG

Rate: Varies from 75-150 per minute during the tracing.
P waves: Neither P waves nor "f" waves are visible.
QRS: Normal.
Conduction: A high percentage of atrial impulses ('f' waves) are blocked at the AV node by
                  the action of digitalis and for this reason the ventricular rate slows.
Rhythm: Irregular throughout.
Comments: Following digitalization the ventricular rate stabilized at 70-80 per minute.

EXAMPLE: **Atrial Fibrillation with a high degree of AV Block**

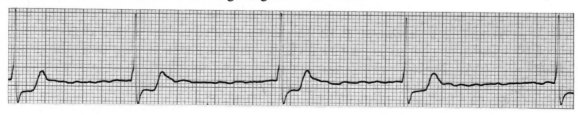

Comments: The very slow ventricular rate (about 50 per minute) is the result of marked AV
                  block due to either excessive amounts of digitalis or damage to the AV node.

CASE HISTORY

A 68-year-old man was admitted to the coronary care unit in acute pulmonary edema. The nurse initiated a planned treatment program which included morphine (15 mg intravenously), rotating tourniquets, the administration of oxygen and an intravenous injection of ethacrynic acid. While there was considerable improvement within the next hour, it was apparent that the left ventricular failure was not fully controlled. The pulse rate was 124 and irregular, and rales were heard throughout the entire chest. The ECG revealed uncontrolled atrial fibrillation. It was felt that the decrease in cardiac output (which produced left ventricular failure) was related in part to the inefficient pumping action associated with atrial fibrillation. On this basis, cardioversion was performed without additional delay. Immediately after the procedure the ventricular rate decreased to 84 per minute and P waves were apparent on the ECG. There was marked improvement in the clinical course thereafter.

EXAMPLE: The Termination of Uncontrolled Atrial Fibrillation by means of Precordial Shock (cardioversion)

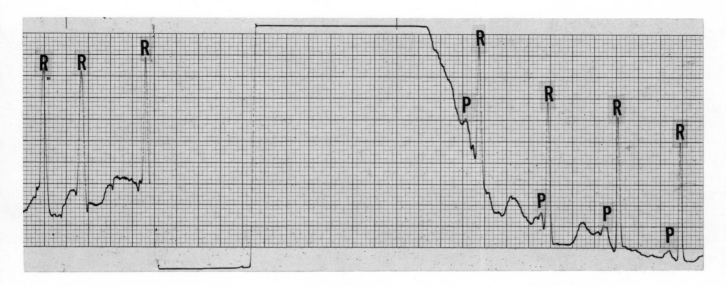

COMMENTS: A precordial shock of 200 watt-seconds (see Chapter 15) was administered to terminate the uncontrolled atrial fibrillation. The effort was successful, as evidenced by the return of normal sinus rythm immediately after the shock.

EXAMPLE: **Atrial Fibrillation — Flutter**

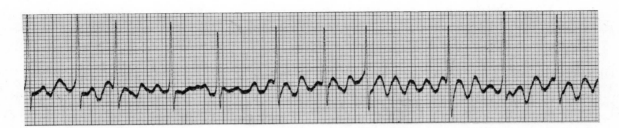

INTERPRETATION OF ECG

Rate: About 110 per minute.

P waves: Not present. There are "saw tooth" F waves of atrial flutter and irregular "f" waves of atrial fibrillation present.

QRS: Normal.

Conduction: Normal beyond the AV node.

Rhythm: Irregular.

Comments: The atrial rhythm vacillates between atrial fibrillation and atrial flutter reflecting the close relationship of these two arrhythmias.

ATRIAL STANDSTILL

ETIOLOGY

The SA node and the entire atrial muscle lose their capacity to generate electrical impulses and the pacemaking function is assumed by the *AV node or the ventricles.* This failure of the *supraventricular* pacemaking centers usually develops in a progressive manner, first with loss of the SA node stimulus and then loss of atrial pacemaking function. This sequence is described as *"downward displacement of the pacemaker"* and is usually a terminal arrhythmia associated with advanced left ventricular failure. Very rarely, this arrhythmia may result from overdosages of digitalis and quinidine, or from electrolyte disturbances.

CLINICAL FEATURES

1. Atrial standstill can only be recognized from the ECG. There are no symptoms or physical findings diagnostic of this arrhythmia.
2. As noted, atrial standstill occurs most often in the setting of advanced left ventricular failure and a rather sudden loss of P waves usually suggests that downward displacement of the pacemaker is occurring.

DANGER IN ACUTE MYOCARDIAL INFARCTION

1. The failure of the SA node and the atria to function leaves the AV node and the ventricles as the only remaining pacemakers. These latter centers are far less dependable than the supraventricular pacemakers, and *ventricular standstill* may occur at any time.
2. "Downward displacement of the pacemaker" usually indicates irreversible damage of the higher pacing centers and heralds death.
3. *RISK:* An extremely ominous arrhythmia and usually an immediate forerunner of death due to advanced left ventricular failure.

TREATMENT

1. If the arrhythmia is due to extensive myocardial damage and progressive tissue ischemia, there is little hope for survival with present therapy. Treatment should be directed primarily to improving left ventricular function.
2. A transvenous pacing catheter should be inserted with the first suspicion that the SA node or atria are failing as pacemakers and ventricular pacing should be carried out during the course of treatment for left ventricular failure.
3. If atrial standstill is a result of digitalis toxicity rather than a reflection of progressive ischemia, rapid treatment for such toxicity should be initiated. Potassium or propranolol can be used for this purpose.

NURSING ROLE

1. The P waves should be examined with particular care in all patients with left ventricular failure. A sudden decrease in their amplitude or shape, or the abrupt disappearance of the P waves in this setting may suggest the onset of atrial standstill.
2. Notify the physician immediately and document the changing ECG pattern with a rhythm strip.
3. Verify the patient's clinical status. Death may occur despite the presence of ventricular complexes seen on the monitor. In the other words, although electrical activity may continue, the myocardium is unable to respond, and its pumping action ceases (power failure.)
4. At the first suggestion of atrial standstill preparations should be made for the insertion of a transvenous pacemaker.
5. If a standby pacemaker is already in place when atrial standstill occurs it should be activated.

ATRIAL STANDSTILL — IDENTIFYING ECG FEATURES

1. **Rate:** The rate is usually slow.
2. **P Waves:** There are no P waves and there is essentially a straight line between QRS complexes.
3. **QRS:** The configuration of this complex depends on the site of pacemaker function. If the ventricle is stimulated from the AV node the QRS complex may be normal. When the pacemaker is within the ventricle the QRS will be widened and distorted.
4. **Conduction:** There is no electrical conduction *above* the acting pacemaker.
5. **Rhythm:** The ventricular rhythm is generally regular except in the dying heart.

EXAMPLE: **Atrial Standstill**

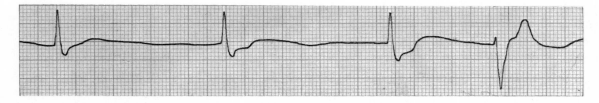

INTERPRETATION OF ECG

Rate:	About 40 per minute.
P waves:	Absent.
QRS:	Widened to 0.12 seconds indicating a delay in ventricular conduction.
Conduction:	The pacemaker has descended to the A-V node.
Rhythm:	Slow and regular.
Comments:	The last complex originated in the ventricle indicating further displacement of the pacemaker.

CASE HISTORY

A 71-year-old man with an acute anteroseptal myocardial infarction was admitted with obvious signs of left ventricular failure. The treatment program included digitalis and a rapid acting diuretic. The response to therapy was poor and the patient remained in heart failure. About eight hours after admission, the nurse noted a change in the previously existing sinus tachycardia. There was a loss of upright P waves along with a decrease in cardiac rate from 128 to 96. The physician was notified immediately. Before his arrival 10 minutes later, the nurse documented a further change in the ECG in the form of inverted P waves (indicating that an atrial pacemaker was now operative). While a transvenous pacemaker was being inserted the rate decreased to 58 and the ECG revealed that all SA and atrial activity had ceased and that the AV node was now the pacemaker. Death occurred despite pacemaking attempts.

The electrocardiographic change from sinus tachycardia (A) to atrial standstill (B) is shown in the following examples:

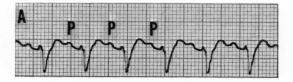

Sinus Tachycardia

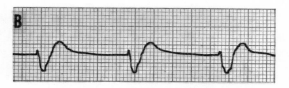

Atrial Standstill

CHAPTER 12

Arrhythmias Originating in the AV Node

There are 2 general types of disorders associated with the AV node. The first is where the AV node *replaces* the SA node as pacemaker (e.g., nodal rhythm or nodal tachycardia). The second is where the AV node *blocks* impulses from the SA node to the ventricles.

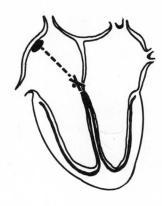

When the cardiac stimulus originates in the *AV node* the impulse is transmitted *downward* in usual fashion through the bundle of His to the ventricles; as a result the QRS complex is normal. The same AV node impulse also extends *upward* to the atria and activates these chambers in reverse order. For this reason, the P waves associated with an AV nodal origin are inverted and may follow the QRS complex.

Under normal conditions the impulse arriving from the SA node is delayed for a fraction of a second before proceeding to the bundle of His; the total time for this conduction is less than 0.20 seconds. When the AV node is damaged, this period of block may be increased with the degree of block depending on the extent of involvement. With minor dysfunction of the AV node the impulse may merely be slowed but then pass through to the ventricle (first degree AV block). If the involvement is more advanced the node may fully block every second, third, or fourth impulse reaching it, causing these impulses to end their journey at this level and never reach the ventricle (second degree AV block). With third degree AV heart block (complete heart block) the node interrupts *all* atrial conduction so that the ventricles beat independently of the atria at their own slow inherent rate. The atria continue to function under the control of the SA node. This means that the atrial and ventricular rates are dissociated and that two independent pacemakers exist.

While AV nodal rhythms probably have the same general significance as atrial arrhythmias their proximity to, and their immediate influence on, ventricular conduction creates additional concern. Rapid rate nodal rhythms (nodal tachycardia) increase the work of the heart and decrease its efficiency.

When the AV node causes heart block the problem is far more serious. This is particularly true in third degree block where the ventricular beat is then dependent on only inherent contractability of the myocardial muscle itself rather than on a more dependable, faster pacemaker. This block may result in ventricular standstill.

Nodal rhythms can be treated with drugs or precordial shock; AV nodal block is usually treated by transvenous pacing. All nodal disturbances should be viewed as *major* arrhythmias.

143

PREMATURE AV NODAL CONTRACTIONS (PNC)

ETIOLOGY

An ectopic stimulus arises *in the AV node* before the onset of the next impulse from the SA node. This stimulus causes a ventricular beat designated as a premature *nodal* contraction (in contrast to a premature ventricular contraction which originates in the ventricle). Irritability of the AV node is the basic source of this ectopic activity.

CLINICAL FEATURES

1. Patients are rarely aware of the presence of premature nodal contractions and symptoms are infrequent.
2. Although some irregularity of the heart beat results from premature nodal contractions (due to the compensatory pause) it is difficult to identify premature nodal contractions specifically by clinical examination and the diagnosis can only be positively established by ECG.

DANGER IN ACUTE MYOCARDIAL INFARCTION

1. Premature nodal contractions are important because they may warn of, and lead to, serious nodal arrhythmias (e.g., nodal tachycardia).
2. An increase in the relative frequency of PNC's can usually be construed as evidence of increasing nodal and myocardial irritability.
3. Infrequent, or isolated, PNC's have no significant effect on circulatory efficiency, and are not of serious consequence in this regard.
4. *RISK:* When PNC's occur infrequently they are not important, but an increase in their frequency may herald serious nodal arrhythmias.

TREATMENT

1. If PNC's occur infrequently, treatment is unnecessary.
2. If their frequency increases, these ectopic beats can usually be terminated by lidocaine or procainamide given intravenously.

NURSING ROLE

1. Identify premature *nodal* contractions and distinguish these from more serious premature *ventricular* contractions.
2. If the relative frequency of PNC's increases, notify the physician.
3. If PNC's are treated by an intravenous infusion of procainamide or lidocaine, the nurse should adjust the rate of flow to control the ectopic beats.

CASE HISTORY

A 58-year-old man with an acute inferior myocardial infarction developed infrequent ectopic beats during the second day of hospitalization. From the monitor lead alone, the nurse was unable to decide whether these beats were premature nodal contractions or premature ventricular contractions. When the frequency of these ectopic beats increased gradually over the next three hours, a 12 lead electrocardiogram was taken to identify this specific origin. Premature nodal contractions were evident. The physician was notified and a lidocaine infusion was started. The ectopic beats disappeared promptly.

PREMATURE AV NODAL CONTRACTIONS (PNC) — IDENTIFYING ECG FEATURES

1. **Rate:** Normal.
2. **P waves:** Because of the origin of impulse in the *AV node*, P waves may not be identified at all; but when visible are either inverted and occur immediately before or after the QRS complex (reflecting their nodal origin).
3. **QRS:** Usually normal but may be wide and aberrant.
4. **Conduction:** The conduction *from* the AV node through the ventricle is normal; however, the conduction between the atria and AV node is retrograde (accounting for P wave changes).
5. **Rhythm:** The rhythm is regular except for the occurrence of the PNC. A compensatory pause (not as long as seen with premature ventricular contractions) creates a minor irregularity of rhythm.

EXAMPLE: **Premature Nodal Contraction**

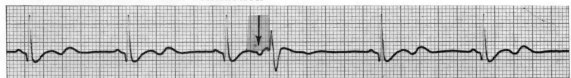

INTERPRETATION OF ECG

Rate: About 55 per minute.

P waves: The P wave of the premature beat is inverted and occurs just before the QRS complex (see arrow).

QRS: The complex is *aberrant* in the premature beat because of the early stimulation of the ventricles (which were not fully recovered from the previous beat).

Conduction: The atria are stimulated in *retrograde* fashion from the AV node in the premature beat.

Rhythm: Regular except for the single ectopic beat.

Comments: The inverted P wave occurring *before* the QRS complex indicates that the impulse originated in the *upper* AV node. If the P wave *followed* the QRS complex, the lower AV node would have been the pacemaker site.

EXAMPLE: **Premature Nodal Contraction**

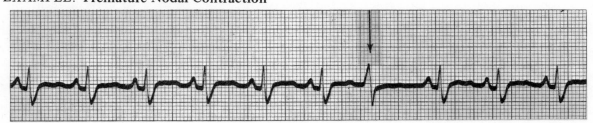

INTERPRETATION OF ECG

Rate: 72 per minute.

P wave: No P wave is found in the premature nodal contraction.

QRS: Normal.

Conduction: Normal from the AV node through the ventricles.

Rhythm: There is a slight delay following the premature beat which creates a minor irregularity in rhythm.

Comments: The absence of the P wave indicates that the premature beat originated in the *middle* of the AV node.

PAROXYSMAL AV NODAL TACHYCARDIA

ETIOLOGY
An irritable center within the *AV node* repeatedly discharges more rapidly than the SA node and assumes the pacemaking role. The impulse spreads downward through the ventricle causing a rapid ventricular response. The arrhythmia usually develops secondary to ischemia of the AV node but digitalis toxicity may occasionally be the underlying cause.

CLINICAL FEATURES
1. The arrhythmia usually begins abruptly, and may terminate with the same suddenness. (This paroxysmal action is similar to that found in paroxysmal atrial tachycardia or in ventricular tachycardia).
2. The symptoms are those anticipated with a rapid ventricular rate. Palpitation and dyspnea are common; and ischemic pain may occur, particularly if the tachycardia is sustained.
3. Paroxysmal nodal tachycardia cannot be distinguished from other regular, rapid rate arrhythmias (e.g., PAT) by clinical examination. The diagnosis can only be established by ECG.

DANGER IN ACUTE MYOCARDIAL INFARCTION
1. The rapid ventricular rate frequently results in a decrease in the cardiac output and predisposes to left ventricular failure as well as myocardial and cerebral ischemia. This threat is related directly to the *duration* of the tachycardia.
2. Nodal tachycardia may deteriorate into ventricular tachycardia or even ventricular fibrillation (indicating that ventricular focus has replaced the AV nodal pacemaker).
3. *RISK:* A very dangerous arrhythmia in terms of hemodynamic consequences and as a warning of impending lethal ventricular arrhythmias.

TREATMENT
1. If nodal tachycardia is *sustained* and results in obvious evidence of circulatory inefficiency (i.e., signs of left ventricular failure, angina, or cerebral ischemia), the arrhythmia should be terminated *immediately* by means of synchronized precordial shock.
2. If the arrhythmia produces no overt symptoms, and the patient is not in distress, drug therapy can be attempted initially. Lidocaine, given intravenously, is the preferred agent.
3. Even if the paroxysm is of short duration and subsides spontaneously without therapy, antiarrhythmic treatment (lidocaine) should nevertheless be instituted to prevent recurrent episodes.
4. If digitalis is suspected as an etiologic factor, the drug should be discontinued. Propranolol or diphenylhydantoin (Dilantin), intravenously, can be used to treat digitalis toxicity.
5. Nodal tachycardia should *not* be allowed to persist under any circumstances and vigorous therapy is indicated to control this arrhythmia.

NURSING ROLE
1. Paroxysmal nodal tachycardia will trigger the high rate alarm system. Identify the presence of this rapid rate arrhythmia and document with ECG strip.
2. Go to the bedside and examine the patient. Assess clinical condition, including respiration, pulse rate, blood pressure, and the presence of symptoms (angina or dyspnea).
3. Notify the physician immediately.
4. Start oxygen therapy.
5. Prepare a syringe containing 100 mg of lidocaine.
6. Prepare for cardioversion.

PAROXYSMAL AV NODAL TACHYCARDIA – IDENTIFYING FEATURES

1. **Rate:** Usually 100-180 per minute.
2. **P waves:** The shape and position of P waves will vary depending on the site of the focus within the AV node. The most likely pattern is an inverted P wave occurring immediately before or after the QRS complex.
3. **QRS:** Normal; conduction beyond the AV node is undisturbed.
4. **Conduction:** The AV node discharges impulses in both directions. Those ascending to the atria cause alterations of the P waves.
5. **Rhythm:** Regular.

EXAMPLE: **AV Nodal Tachycardia**

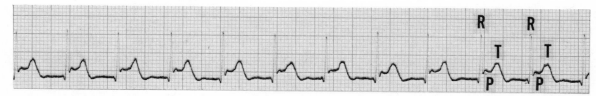

INTERPRETATION OF ECG

Rate: About 110 per minute.
P waves: Inverted and follow the QRS complexes.
QRS: Normal.
Conduction: The ventricle is stimulated by a rapid focus within the AV node; this pacemaker also activates the atria.
Rhythm: Regular.
Comments: This arrhythmia began abruptly and ended spontaneously two minutes later in typical paroxysmal fashion.

EXAMPLE: **Paroxysmal Nodal Tachycardia**

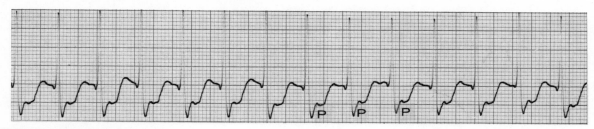

INTERPRETATION OF ECG

Rate: About 140 per minute.
P waves: Follow the QRS complexes.
QRS: Normal.
Conduction: The AV node is the pacemaker for both the atria and ventricles.
Rhythm: Regular.
Comments: It is often difficult to distinguish nodal tachycardia from atrial tachycardia on a single monitor lead and a 12 lead ECG is necessary to identify the presence and position of P waves.

CASE HISTORY

A 50-year-old male with an acute inferior myocardial infarction showed no complications during the first 12 hours after admission. Ten minutes after his lunch, the high rate alarm sounded. The nurse noted a rate of 140 per minute. The monitor showed regular QRS complexes followed by inverted P waves. At the bedside, the nurse observed that the respirations were rapid and that the patient was apprehensive. The blood pressure was 90/60. Oxygen was started and the physician notified. Physical examination by the physician showed signs of early left ventricular failure. An intravenous injection of 100 mg. lidocaine was given rapidly and within 1 minute normal sinus rhythm had returned. A continuous intravenous infusion of lidocaine was then administered to prevent recurrences of the arrhythmia.

AV NODAL RHYTHM

ETIOLOGY

The *AV node* replaces the SA node as the cardiac pacemaker. This displacement results from depression of the SA node permitting the AV node to assume command. (The inherent rhythmicity of the AV node is normally slower than that of the SA node and the AV node does not serve as pacemaker *unless* the rate of the SA node is markedly depressed.)

Impulses from the AV node spread both *downward* to the ventricles and *upward* to the atria. Thus, with AV nodal rhythm the AV node controls both atrial and ventricular activity. The depression of the SA node which causes nodal rhythm is usually the result of excessive vagal activity. Ischemic damage of the SA node or digitalis toxicity are other causative factors.

CLINICAL FEATURES

1. This arrhythmia seldom produces symptoms.
2. The only clinical finding suggesting AV nodal rhythm is a slow, *regular* rate, usually between 40 and 60 beats per minute.
3. AV nodal rhythm cannot be distinguished with certainty from other bradycardias except by ECG.
4. AV nodal rhythm is often temporary and the SA node may regain its normal role spontaneously.

DANGER IN ACUTE MYOCARDIAL INFARCTION

1. Because of the inherently slow rate of nodal impulses, ectopic foci with more rapid rates may take over the pacemaking function. Such foci may cause either nodal or ventricular tachycardia.
2. Nodal rhythm may lead to complete heart block or ventricular standstill.
3. As with other slow rate arrhythmias cardiac output may be decreased and cause cerebral or myocardial insufficiency.
4. *RISK:* While seldom dangerous in its own right, AV nodal rhythm indicates a less-dependable pacemaker than the SA node is in command and poses the potential threat of more serious ectopic rhythms developing.

TREATMENT

1. There is no specific drug therapy for AV nodal rhythm.
2. If the slow heart rate compromises the circulation, a transvenous pacemaker can be used to increase the ventricular rate (See Chapter 15).
3. If ventricular ectopic beats develop in the presence of AV nodal rhythm, lidocaine should be used to control the irritable ventricle.
4. If the arrhythmia is secondary to overdosages of digitalis, or quinidine, the offending drug should be withdrawn promptly.

NURSING ROLE

1. Identify the arrhythmia as a nodal rhythm; rule out sinus bradycardia and advanced heart block as causes of this slow rate.
2. Observe the monitor carefully for premature ventricular contractions or other ectopic activity, developing in the presence of a nodal rhythm. Notify the physician if such ectopic activity is noted.
3. When the rate is below 50, be particularly alert for signs of decreased cardiac efficiency.
4. If nodal rhythm suddenly develops, notify the physician.
5. Among patients receiving digitalis or quinidine discuss further administration of these drugs with the physician.

AV NODAL RHYTHM — IDENTIFYING ECG FEATURES

1. **Rate:** Slow, usually between 40 and 60 per minute.
2. **P waves:** Abnormal; usually inverted. They may occur a) *before* the QRS (upper nodal), b) *after* the QRS (lower nodal), or c) may not be visible, being buried within the QRS (middle nodal).
3. **QRS:** Normal.
4. **Conduction:** The conduction *downward* through the ventricular pathways is normal resulting in an undisturbed QRS complex. The atria are stimulated in a retrograde fashion accounting for the inversion of the P waves.
5. **Rhythm:** Regular.

EXAMPLE: **AV Nodal Rhythm**

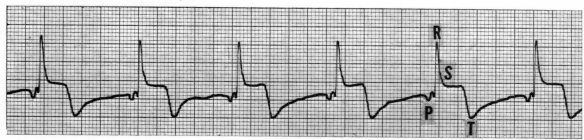

INTERPRETATION OF ECG

Rate: About 58 per minute.

P waves: Inverted and occur .06 seconds before the QRS complex characteristic of upper nodal rhythm.

QRS: Normal.

Conduction: The AV is the pacemaker. The impulse passes downward through the ventricular pathway and upward to the atria.

Rhythm: Regular.

Comments: The ST segment elevations and T wave inversions are characteristic of acute myocardial infarction.

EXAMPLE: **AV Nodal Rhythm**

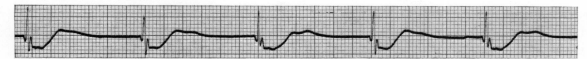

INTERPRETATION OF ECG

Rate: About 50 per minute.

P waves: Not specifically identified being lost within the QRS complex (middle nodal rhythm).

QRS: Normal.

Conduction: Normal below the AV node.

Rhythm: Regular.

Comments: The slow regular rate is characteristic of an AV nodal pacemaker.

CASE HISTORY

A 52-year-old man was admitted to the CCU with a heart rate of 52 per minute. He was in no distress and there was no evidence of circulatory failure. The nurse recognized the cause of this bradycardia as a lower nodal rhythm on the basis of inverted P waves which followed the QRS complexes.

Two hours after being examined by the physician, the patient developed premature *ventricular* contractions which occurred at a rate of 1-2 per minute. Recognizing the potential danger of these ectopic beats, the nurse notified the physician. Lidocaine was given by intravenous infusion and the ectopic beats were controlled promptly. Three days later the nodal rhythm disappeared and a normal sinus rhythm returned.

DELAYED AV CONDUCTION (FIRST DEGREE HEART BLOCK)

ETIOLOGY

The impulse arises in the *SA node* and is conducted normally to the AV node. Within the AV node the impulse is abnormally *delayed* (prolonged PR interval) before its passage to the ventricular conduction system. This delay usually results from ischemia of the AV node, but drugs may also produce this block in conduction.

CLINICAL FEATURES

1. There are no symptoms or physical findings characteristic of first degree AV block.
2. The diagnosis can *only* be made by ECG.

DANGER IN MYOCARDIAL INFARCTION

1. First degree AV block is not a serious arrhythmia in its own right. It does not reduce the hemodynamic efficiency nor does it affect the rate or rhythm of the heart.
2. The arrhythmia is important because it reflects injury of the AV node and may warn of impending second or third degree heart blocks. These latter blocks, which are *advanced* stages of AV nodal involvement, are extremely dangerous and may lead to ventricular standstill.
3. *RISK:* Often an early warning of more advanced heart block, but not a dangerous arrhythmia in itself.

TREATMENT

1. If the delay in conduction is moderate (PR interval of 0.21 to 0.25), and does not increase, treatment is unnecessary.
2. If the conduction delay is greater than 0.26 sec., or if it increases, atropine, 1 mg. intravenously should be used in an attempt to decrease the degree of AV block. However, the drug is not predictably effective in this purpose, and isoproterenol can be used in the event of failure with atropine.
3. If drug therapy is unsuccessful in controlling a *progressive* first degree block, the insertion of a transvenous pacing catheter is frequently indicated on a "standby" basis. This prophylactic approach reduces the risk of rapid *unpredictable* progression of first degree block to complete block or ventricular standstill.
4. If first degree heart block develops during the course of treatment with digitalis or any antiarrhythmic agent, the further use of these drugs should be carefully considered in view of their known ability to depress the AV node.

NURSING ROLE

1. When first degree heart block is identified, carefully measure the PR interval. If the PR interval is greater than 0.26 seconds or if it shows progressive lengthening subsequently, the physician should be notified.
2. Carefully observe the monitor for the sudden appearance of second or third degree heart block. If such advanced heart block develops, notify the physician *immediately.*
3. Among patients agents receiving digitalis or other anti-arrhythmic agents discuss the further administration of these drugs with the physician.

DELAYED AV CONDUCTION (FIRST DEGREE HEART BLOCK)
IDENTIFYING ECG FEATURES

1. **Rate:**   Normal.
2. **P waves:**   Normal, since P waves originate in the SA node.
3. **QRS:**   Normal.
4. **Conduction:** PR interval is *prolonged* beyond .20 seconds. This is the only abnormality. Ventricular conduction is normal.
5. **Rhythm:**   Regular.

EXAMPLE: **First Degree AV Block**

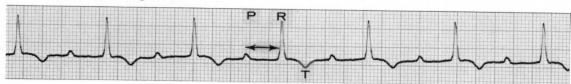

INTERPRETATION OF ECG

Rate: About 65 per minute.

P waves: Normal.

QRS: Normal.

Conduction: The PR interval is almost .40 seconds indicating a conduction delay through the AV node.

Rhythm: Regular.

Comments: Marked first degree block of this type may progress to more advanced AV block.

EXAMPLE: **First Degree AV Block**

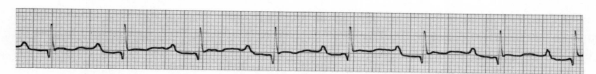

INTERPRETATION OF ECG

Rate: About 75 per minute.

P waves: Normal.

QRS: Normal.

Conduction: The PR conduction is about .32 seconds. Subsequent conduction is normal.

Rhythm: Regular.

Comments: Atropine will often decrease the AV block and the PR interval may become normal.

CASE HISTORY

A 46-year-old man with an acute inferior myocardial infarction had evidence of a first degree heart block at the time of his admission. On the admission rhythm strip the nurse noted a PR interval of 0.22 seconds. Eight hours later, the PR interval measured 0.28 seconds and the physician was notified immediately. Atropine was given intravenously, but its effectiveness was short lived, and within one hour the PR interval had increased additionally to 0.30 seconds. The physician was advised again and an infusion of isoproterenol was ordered. The response was excellent and the PR interval returned to normal very promptly.

SECOND DEGREE AV HEART BLOCK

ETIOLOGY

The impulse, originating in the *SA node*, reaches the AV node in normal fashion, but the AV node then blocks every second, third or fourth impulse from reaching the ventricular conduction system. Thus, there is only one ventricular beat for every two, three, or four atrial impulses; this discrepancy in rates is described as 2:1, 3:1, or 4:1 AV block. This type of block results most often from ischemic damage to the AV node. Digitalis can also cause second degree block.

CLINICAL FEATURES

1. Unless the ventricular rate is markedly slow, the patient may remain unaware of the presence of this arrhythmia. However, if the block occurs *suddenly*, some patients may recognize the abrupt change in rate.
2. The diagnosis of second degree AV block is made primarily with an ECG.

DANGER IN MYOCARDIAL INFARCTION

1. Second degree block usually indicates serious involvement of the AV node. Patients with second degree AV block are high-risk candidates for complete (3rd degree) AV block. This progression, or advancement, may occur with distressing rapidity.
2. The reduced ventricular rate associated with second degree block may adversely affect circulatory efficiency, but such impairment is unusual and 2:1 and 3:1 blocks are most often tolerated well.
3. Second degree AV block is often a *temporary* disturbance with acute myocardial infarction and usually subsides within 72 to 96 hours.
4. *RISK:* An important, and potentially dangerous, arrhythmia. Second degree block must be viewed as a *warning* arrhythmia preceding complete heart block and ventricular standstill.

TREATMENT

1. Because of the *unpredictable* course of second degree block, and the ever-present threat of sudden advancement to complete block or ventricular standstill, it is good practice to position a transvenous pacemaker catheter in the right ventricle, as soon as this arrhythmia is identified. If the ventricular rate is below 60 per minute, pacing should be initiated. When the ventricular rate is more rapid, the pacemaker can be kept on a "standby" basis. (See Chapter 15)
2. There is no sure means for increasing conduction through the AV node but isoproterenol (Isuprel) is often effective in this purpose and an intravenous infusion of this drug (1 mg in 250 cc of 5% D/W solution) can be attempted while preparing for transvenous pacemaker insertion. Atropine, given intravenously (1 mg), sometimes decreases the degree of AV block but is less effective than isoproterenol.
3. With the slim hope that second degree block has been caused by digitalis or quinidine, these drugs should be *withdrawn* in the presence of advanced block.
4. On the premise that the AV node and conduction system are affected by myocardial edema, corticosteroid therapy is occasionally used and may be successful.

NURSING ROLE

1. Identify the slow rate arrhythmia as second degree block and document the disturbance on a rhythm strip. Second degree block must be distinguished from sinus bradycardia or third degree (complete) AV block.
2. Notify the physician promptly as soon as second degree block is identified.
3. Prepare for the insertion of a transvenous pacemaker.
4. Prepare an infusion containing 1 mg of isoproterenol in 250 cc of 5% D/W solution. (Microdrip administration and the use of "piggyback" technique is essential.)
5. If second degree block is present, further doses of digitalis and antiarrhythmic agents should be withheld until the physician has assessed the problem.
6. Observe the monitor carefully for progression of the degree of block. *Remember* that third degree block or ventricular standstill may be only a step behind.

SECOND DEGREE AV HEART BLOCK – IDENTIFYING ECG FEATURES

1. **Rate:** The ventricular rate is usually slow and is one-half, or one-third, or one-quarter of the atrial rate.
2. **P waves:** There are two, three, or four times as many P waves as QRS complexes.
3. **QRS:** Normal.
4. **Conduction:** Every second, third, or fourth beat coming to the AV node is *blocked* and never reaches the ventricular conduction system.
5. **Rhythm:** Slow and regular.

EXAMPLE: **Second Degree AV Block**

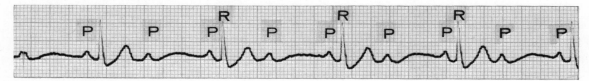

INTERPRETATION OF ECG

Rate: Ventricular rate 47 per minute. Atrial rate 94 per minute.

P waves: There are two normal P waves between ventricular complexes.

QRS: Normal.

Conduction: Alternate P waves are blocked at the AV node. Conduction proceeds normally to the ventricles from those impulses that pass through the node.

Rhythm: Regular.

Comments: The ventricular rate is one half the atrial rate (2:1 block).

EXAMPLE: **Second Degree AV Block (Wenckebach type)**

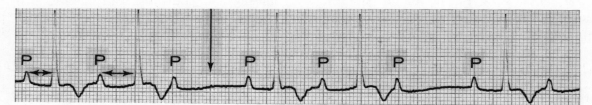

Comments: Unlike the first example in which every *other* atrial impulse was blocked *regularly* in the AV node, this tracing shows AV block which occurs *irregularly*. This latter type of second degree block is called the *Wenckebach Phenomenon*. It reflects *progressive* difficulty of conduction through the AV node. The sequence begins with a prolonged PR interval (see first complex) which progresses in duration (see second complex) until the atrial impulse is blocked completely (see arrow) so that a QRS complex fails to occur. Following the dropped QRS complex the sequence is repeated. Thus, in this example, every third atrial impulse is blocked creating an irregular ventricular response.

CASE HISTORY

A 72-year-old man with an acute inferior myocardial infarction was admitted to the C C U in no distress. His pulse rate originally was 78 per minute. Two hours later the low rate alarm sounded when the pulse fell to 52 per minute. The nurse recognized second degree AV block and obtained a rhythm strip documenting the arrhythmia. She notified the physician of the sudden occurrence of this block, and was instructed to prepare an infusion of isoproterenol. One hour after the start of this therapy, it was apparent that second degree block was still present and the physician was notified again. A temporary transvenous pacing catheter was then positioned in the right ventricle by the physician. This was attached to a demand pacemaker, which would initiate pacing whenever the heart rate fell below 60 per minute. Within 72 hours, a normal sinus rhythm had returned, and the pacing catheter was removed.

COMPLETE AV HEART BLOCK (THIRD DEGREE BLOCK)

ETIOLOGY

The AV node blocks *all* impulse from the SA node; as a consequence the atria and ventricles beat *independently*. The SA node serves as the pacemaker for the atria while the ventricles contract with the inherent rhythmicity of ventricular tissue at a rate of 25-40 beats per minute.

The most common cause of complete heart block is ischemic damage to the AV node. Rarely, extreme digitalis toxicity may be responsible for the block.

CLINICAL FEATURES

1. The ventricles beat at a regular, *fixed* rate, usually less than 40 per minute. (This clinical finding by itself should be cause for suspicion of the presence of complete heart block.)
2. Cerebral ischemia manifested by syncope (Stokes-Adams attacks), is common in the presence of third degree block and results from decreased cardiac output secondary to the very slow ventricular rate.
3. Signs and symptoms of left ventricular failure are frequently present.

DANGER IN ACUTE MYOCARDIAL INFARCTION

1. The *independent* ventricular pacemaker is not dependable and may cease abruptly (ventricular standstill), or may be replaced by a faster irritable focus in the ventricle (leading to ventricular tachycardia or ventricular fibrillation).
2. Because the ventricular rate is *fixed* at 30-40 beats per minute and cannot increase to meet circulatory demands, the cardiac output is inadequate in most instances which predisposes to left ventricular failure.
3. Reduced blood flow to the brain may result in fainting and convulsions (Stokes-Adams syndrome). Lesser degrees of cerebral blood flow impairment are manifested by mental confusion and vertigo.
4. *RISK:* An *extremely* dangerous arrhythmia representing a clear warning of impending ventricular standstill, ventricular fibrillation, and left ventricular failure.

TREATMENT

1. The most dependable and predictably effective method of treating complete heart block is transvenous cardiac pacing. A catheter electrode should be positioned in the right ventricle as soon as third degree block is identified.
2. While preparing for the insertion of a pacemaker, an intravenous infusion of isoproterenol (1mg in 250 cc of glucose solution) should be administered. On some occasions, the isoproterenol may reduce the degree of AV block and increase the heart rate. Despite this seeming effectiveness, sudden recurrence of complete block often occurs with drug therapy and it is a wise practice to insert a transvenous pacemaker in *all* patients who develop complete heart block.
3. Transvenous pacing should be continued until normal sinus rhythm returns and the pacing catheter should remain in place on a standby basis for at least five days thereafter.
4. Rarely, complete heart block persists because of *irreversible* damage to the AV node. In this circumstance a permanent pacemaker will be required.
5. Because complete heart block is frequently preceded by lesser degrees of AV block the treatment of this arrhythmia ideally should begin when progressive heart block is first identified. This implies that a transvenous pacemaker should be inserted when second degree heart block is present, as a prophylactic measure.

> ## COMPLETE AV HEART BLOCK (THIRD DEGREE BLOCK)
> ### IDENTIFYING ECG FEATURES
>
> 1. **Rate:** The ventricular rate is usually *less* than 40 per minute and more often near 30. The atrial rate is usually normal.
> 2. **P waves:** There are more P waves than QRS complexes. The size and shape of the P waves are normal.
> 3. **QRS:** Configuration of the complex depends on the site of the ectopic ventricular pacemaker. May be normal if impulse originates close to the AV node.
> 4. **Conduction:** There are 2 separate pacemakers with no relationship between atrial and ventricular rhythms. There is no conduction across the AV node.
> 5. **Rhythm:** Both atrial and ventricular rhythms are regular; although, totally independent of each other.

EXAMPLE: **Complete Heart Block (Third Degree Block)**

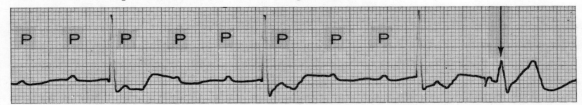

INTERPRETATION OF ECG

Rate: The ventricular rate is 37 per minute. The atrial rate is about 110 per minute.

P waves: Occur regularly but independent of the QRS complexes.

QRS: Normal.

Conduction: There is no conduction between the atria and ventricles; each functioning under the control of its own pacemaker.

Rhythm: The atrial and ventricular rhythms are both regular.

Comments: A premature ventricular contraction (see arrow) is seen at the end of the tracing. Because of the very slow ventricular rate ectopic foci of this type are common with complete heart block and create a risk of ventricular tachycardia and fibrillation.

NURSING ROLE

1. Identify this slow rate arrhythmia and distinguish it from marked sinus bradycardia, nodal rhythm and from second degree AV block. Document with a rhythm strip.
2. Notify the physician *immediately* after this arrhythmia is recognized.
3. Prepare an infusion containing 1 mg of isoproterenol in 250 cc of dextrose solution.
4. Because of the threat of ventricular fibrillation developing in the presence of this slow rate arrhythmia, the defibrillator should be brought to the bedside and made ready for use.
5. A syringe containing 100 mg of lidocaine should be prepared and kept at the bedside.
6. Preparation should be made for the insertion of a transvenous pacemaker , (See Chapter 15)
7. Assess the patient's clinical condition on a continuous basis with particular emphasis on the development of signs or symptoms of left ventricular failure.
8. Diligently seek premature ventricular contractions on the monitor, since these ectopic beats may forewarn of the development of ventricular tachycardia or fibrillation.
9. If a transvenous pacemaker had been inserted *previously* because of advancing, but lesser degrees, of AV block, and is on a standby basis, the nurse should turn on the pacemaker at the first sign of complete heart block. (If a demand pacemaker is used, manual activation by the nurse is unnecessary. Nevertheless, effective pacing function should be verified.)
10. If the patient develops ventricular standstill *before* a pacemaker has been inserted, initiate the planned program for resuscitation (including external pacing) as described in Chapter 15.

Three Examples of Complete Heart Block

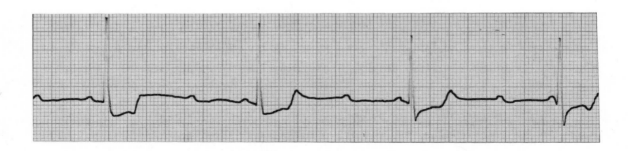

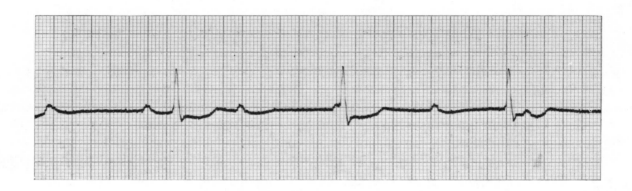

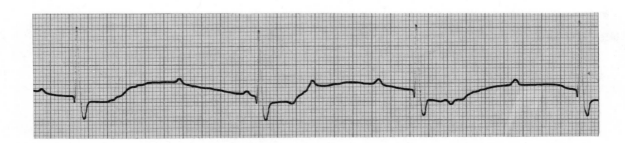

Comments:	These three examples show the typical electrocardiographic patterns of complete (3rd degree) AV heart block. Note the following key identifying features:
Rate:	In each instance the ventricular rate is less than 40 per minute (the inherent rhythmic rate of ventricular muscle).
P waves:	The atrial rate is more rapid than the ventricular rate and the P waves are unrelated to the QRS complexes. The P-R interval is inconstant.(This one feature offers an immediate clue to the diagnosis).

CASE HISTORY

A 58-year-old man was admitted to the coronary care unit with a second degree AV heart block. He was not in acute distress. His blood pressure was 136/90 and the pulse was 54 per minute. The physician was notified of these admission findings and plans were made for the insertion of a transvenous pacemaker within an hours time. During preparations for this procedure the low rate alarm sounded. The nurse recognized that a complete heart block had developed. On examining the patient she found the pulse to be 34 per minute, and the blood pressure 96/80. The patient complained of recurrent chest pain and dyspnea. An infusion of isoproterenol was started immediately and continued until a transvenous pacemaker was inserted and functioning properly. When the heart was paced at a rate of 60 per minute there was marked clinical improvement. (See example below).

EXAMPLE: **Case History**

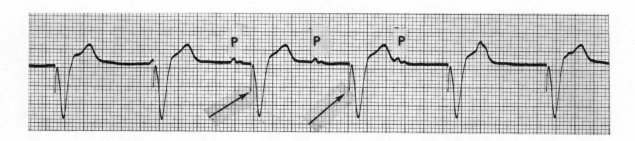

Comments: Although the complete heart block still exists (as evidenced by the random positions of the P waves), the ventricular rate is now controlled by the pacemaker. The pacing stimulus (see arrows) occurs at a rate of about 60 per minute creating a ventricular response at this rate.

EXAMPLE: **Complete Heart Block leading to Ventricular Tachycardia and Fibrillation**

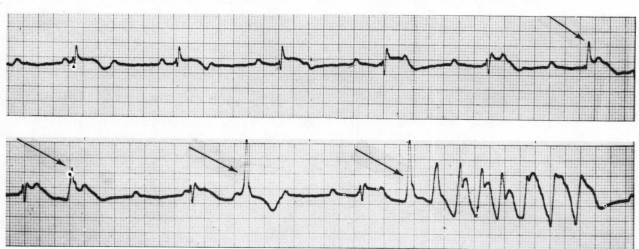

Comments: The electrocardiographic sequence shown above demonstrates one of the great dangers of complete heart block: *ventricular fibrillation.* In the presence of the very slow ventricular rate associated with complete heart block, premature ventricular contractions developed (see arrows). These ectopic beats resulted in ventricular tachycardia and fibrillation (see lower ECG strip). The basis of this complication is described in the following section on ventricular arrhythmias.

CHAPTER 13

Arrhythmias Originating in the Ventricles

Disturbances in the heart beat that originate in the SA node, the atria, or the AV node are jointly classified as *supraventricular* arrhythmias. If the impulse begins in the ventricles, below the level of the AV node, the resulting disorder is termed a *ventricular* arrhythmia.

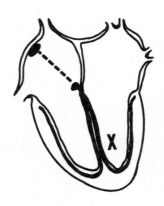

There are three general groups of ventricular arrhythmias: a) those resulting from irritability of the ventricles as manifest by premature ventricular contractions; b) those resulting from damage to the ventricular conducting pathway (bundle branch block); or c) those which cause sudden death (i.e., ventricular fibrillation and ventricular standstill). This last category is considered separately in the next chapter.

The most common ventricular arrhythmia (in fact the most common of *all* arrhythmias) is the premature ventricular contraction. This results from the discharge of an ectopic focus, within the ventricular walls or conducting pathway before the expected arrival of the next impulse from the atria. These premature beats reflect irritability of the ventricles and their rate of occurrence is probably a fair index of the degree of such irritation.

There is now strong evidence that ventricular fibrillation is a direct consequence of myocardial irritability and that this lethal arrhythmia usually begins with a premature ventricular contraction. The scale of irritability leading to ventricular fibrillation can be viewed as follows:

a) occasional premature ventricular contractions.

b) premature ventricular contractions occurring more than six times a minute or originating from different ventricular foci (multifocal premature beats).

c) a series of consecutive premature ventricular contractions (ventricular tachycardia).

d) ventricular fibrillation.

With a few exceptions, ventricular arrhythmias are more significant and more serious than the supraventricular types, since it is not the atrial activity but the ventricular response of an arrhythmia that determines its prognosis. For instance in atrial flutter where the atria contact 200-400 times each minute the circulation may not be endangered because the AV node blocks at least half of these impulses and the ventricles are protected accordingly. In contrast, with ventricular arrhythmias (e.g., ventricular tachycardia) the effect of the disturbance is manifest directly on the output of the heart and the risk is much greater.

It is now quite clear that premature ventricular contractions should be treated vigorously and not allowed to persist, unless they are very infrequent, if ventricular fibrillation is to be prevented. Lidocaine has become the drug of choice for this purpose. Ventricular tachycardia is frequently an immediate forerunner of ventricular fibrillation and demands emergency treatment. This arrhythmia may be terminated with either lidocaine or precordial shock.

PREMATURE VENTRICULAR CONTRACTIONS

ETIOLOGY

An irritable focus within the ventricle discharges *before* the SA node initiates the next anticipated impulse. This ectopic focus stimulates the ventricle directly and causes a *premature ventricular contraction.* Premature ventricular contractions are the most common of all arrhythmias associated with acute myocardial infarction and are a sign of ventricular irritability.

CLINICAL FEATURES

1. Most patients recognize premature beats and describe the sensation as "palpitation" or "my heart is skipping." Awareness of this irregularity in rhythm can usually be correlated with the frequency of these ectopic beats.
2. When listening to the heart, or taking the pulse, a long pause is noted immediately after the premature beat. This delay (called the compensatory pause) is characteristic of premature ventricular contractions and is practically diagnostic of this arrhythmia.

DANGER IN ACUTE MYOCARDIAL INFARCTION

1. Premature ventricular contractions reflect myocardial irritability and, as such, warn of ventricular tachycardia and ventricular fibrillation.
   Premature ventricular contractions are particularly dangerous if they exist in any of the four following forms:
   a) when PVC^s occur frequently, six or more times per minute.
   b) when every second beat is a PVC (bigeminy).
   c) when the premature ventricular contraction strikes near, or on the T wave of the preceding complex (the "R on T" pattern).
   d) when premature ventricular contractions originate from more than one irritable focus (multifocal PVC^s).
2. Premature ventricular contractions occur in about 80% of all patients with acute myocardial infarction. An increase in their frequency is more significant than merely their presence.
3. Overdosages of digitalis often cause PVC^s. This relationship is suggested especially when PVC^s occur as bigeminy.
4. *RISK:* If PVC^s are isolated, or occur infrequently, they seldom pose a serious threat. However, if these ectopic beats occur with increasing frequency, or are multifocal in origin, they should be considered as a serious *warning* of impending ventricular tachycardia or ventricular fibrillation.

TREATMENT

1. *Lidocaine* is the primary agent for treating PVC^s. For quick control of the irritable focus the drug is administered as a rapid, intravenous injection ("push-dose") of 50-100 mg. This should be followed by a continuous infusion of lidocaine given at a rate of 1 mg per minute (10 microdrops of a solution containing 1,000 mg in 250 cc of glucose solution) to suppress further irritability. Procainamide (Pronestyl) can be used intravenously instead of lidocaine, but has the disadvantage of producing hypotension and for this reason is a less desirable choice.
2. If lidocaine (or procainamide) fail to suppress PVC^s an intravenous infusion of potassium (40 mEg. KCl in 500 cc dextrose solution) is effective very often and should be used in this circumstance.
3. Premature ventricular beats can sometimes be abolished with anti-arrhythmic agents administered *orally.* Procainamide, in dosages of 500 mg every 6 hours, or quinidine (400 mg every 6 hours), are the most effective of the oral agents. Because of their slow action these drugs should not be used for immediate control of dangerous forms of PVC^s.
4. If PVC^s are infrequent, but cause apprehension to the patient, sedatives or tranquilizers can be given.
5. If PVC^s develop during treatment with digitalis, the possibility of digitalis toxicity should always be considered.

PREMATURE VENTRICULAR CONTRACTIONS – IDENTIFYING ECG FEATURES

1. **Rate:** Usually normal, but PVCˢ can occur at any rate.
2. **P waves:** Not identifiable in the ectopic beat because the impulse originates in the ventricle and not in the SA node or atrium.
3. **QRS:** *Always* widened and distorted in shape. The configuration of QRS complex depends on the site of the ventricular stimulus.
4. **Conduction:** The ventricle is stimulated directly and there is no conduction from the atrium to the ventricle for the isolated PVC. The beats preceding and following the PVC show normal PQRST complexes.
5. **Rhythm:** The time between the beat preceding and the beat following the PVC is equal to two normal beats (compensatory pause).

EXAMPLE: **Isolated Premature Ventricular Contraction**

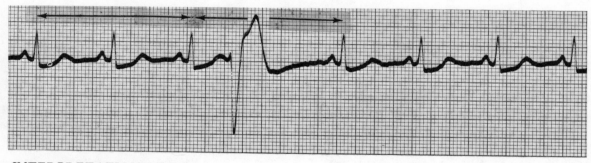

INTERPRETATION OF ECG

Rate: 74 per minute.

P waves: Absent in premature contraction; otherwise normal.

QRS: The ectopic complex is widened and bizarre in configuration and the T wave is oppositely directed to the QRS complex.

Conduction: The impulse for the PVC originates in the ventricle. The conduction of the remaining beats is normal.

Rhythm: Regular except for PVC.

Comments: The interval between the beat preceding the PVC and the beat following the PVC is equal to the time of two normal beats (see arrows).

NURSING ROLE

1. Identify premature ventricular contractions and distinguish these ectopic beats from atrial or nodal premature contractions.
2. Carefully assess the relative frequency of PVCˢ during successive time intervals to ascertain any change.
3. If PVCˢ occur in any of the most threatening forms, the physician should be notified and lidocaine prepared for immediate administration.
4. If an infusion of lidocaine is used to control PVCˢ, adjust the rate of flow to continuously suppress ectopic activity.
5. If lidocaine is given repeatedly or in large quantities, seek signs of overdosage as manifested by petit mal, or rarely, grand mal seizures. If procainamide is being used instead of lidocaine, drug-induced hypotension should be carefully sought.
6. In the event PVCˢ develop during digitalis therapy, advise the physician before administering the next dose of digitalis.

DANGEROUS FORMS OF PREMATURE VENTRICULAR CONTRACTIONS

1. Frequent PVC^S occurring more than six per minute.

EXAMPLE:

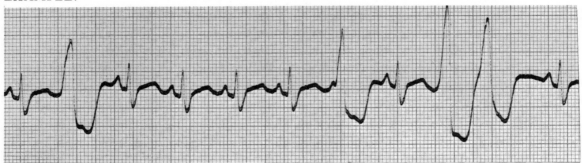

INTERPRETATION OF ECG

Rate: About 80 per minute.

P waves: Not identified in ectopic beats.

QRS: The ectopic beats are widened and distorted in shape.

Conduction: The premature beats originate in tne ventricle; the remaining beats are conducted normally from the SA node.

Rhythm: Irregular because of premature beats.

Comments: There are four PVC^S within this six second strip. Two of them are consecutive. This high frequency of PVC^S indicates marked ventricular irritability.

2. Bigeminy (alternate PVC^S or coupled rhythm).

EXAMPLE:

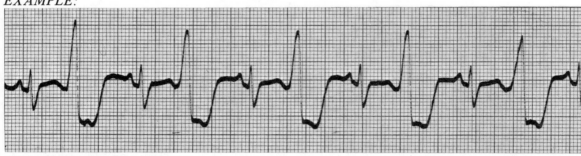

INTERPRETATION OF ECG

Rate: About 100 per minute.

P waves: The P waves are absent in the PVC^S.

QRS: Grossly distorted and obviously different from the beats originating in the SA node.

Conduction: The ventricle is stimulated directly by an ectopic focus within the ventricular wall in every other complex.

Rhythm: Irregular due to coupled beats.

Comments: Bigeminy is often an immediate forerunner of ventricular tachycardia and warns of this more dangerous arrhythmia.

CASE HISTORY

A 51-year-old woman with an acute myocardial infarction showed evidence of PVC^S from the time of her admission to the unit. These ectopic beats occurred at a rate 1-2 per minute. During the next several hours, the nurse noted the PVC^S gradually increased in frequency and that bigeminy had developed. The physician was advised of this change and a "push dose" of lidocaine (75 mg) was given. The PVC^S disappeared within a minute of the injection. An intravenous infusion of lidocaine was then started. Two hours later, the PVC^S reappeared and the nurse increased the rate of infusion from 1 mg to 2 mgs per minute after which the PVC^S disappeared.

3. The R on T Pattern

EXAMPLE:

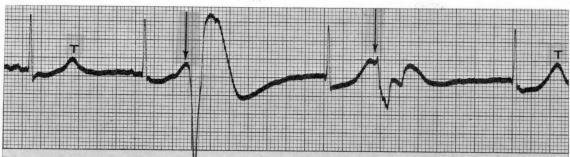

INTERPRETATION OF ECG

Rate: About 60 per minute.
P waves: Not present in premature ventricular contraction.
QRS: The two ectopic beats are both distorted and have different configurations.
Conduction: The ectopic beats arise in the ventricle. The difference in their configuration indicates that more than one irritable focus is present in the ventricle.
Rhythm: The ectopic beats create an irregularity in the basic rhythm.
Comments: Both premature ventricular contractions strike *directly* on the T waves of the preceding complexes (see arrows). This relationship of the PVC to the T wave (R on T pattern) predisposes to the onset of ventricular fibrillation as shown in the following example:

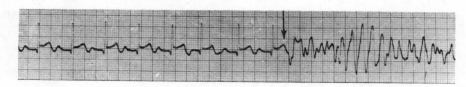

4. Multifocal PVC^S

EXAMPLE:

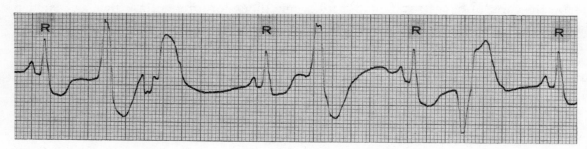

INTERPRETATION OF ECG

Rate: About 75 per minute.
P waves: There are no P waves with the PVC[S].
QRS: All of the premature beats have widened and distorted QRS complexes; but these vary in contour from each other since they originate from separate ventricular foci (multifocal PVC[S]).
Conduction: There is no conduction from the atria to the ventricles in the premature beats.
Rhythm: Irregular.
Comments: Multifocal PVC[S] reflect advanced ventricular irritability and vigorous antiarrhythmic treatment must be used to terminate this ectopic activity.

VENTRICULAR TACHYCARDIA

ETIOLOGY

Ventricular tachycardia can be defined as four or more *consecutive* premature ventricular contractions. These repetitive premature beats reflect advanced myocardial irritability and indicate that a persistent ectopic focus in the ventricular wall commands the heart rate.

Ventricular tachycardia may occasionally develop spontaneously, but usually there is preceding evidence of ventricular irritability in the form of premature ventricular contractions. When these ectopic beats occur *repetitively,* ventricular tachycardia exists. Because ventricular tachycardia represents advanced myocardial irritability it must be recognized as an immediate forerunner of *ventricular fibrillation.*

CLINICAL FEATURES

1. Most patients are immediately aware of the sudden onset of rapid heart action and describe palpitation and dyspnea. When these latter symptoms are associated with chest pain (a common situation) the patient often suspects that a castastrophic event has occurred and marked apprehension is immediately evident.
2. The blood pressure generally falls after the onset of this arrhythmia, and findings of left ventricular failure may develop with surprising rapidity if the tachycardia is sustained.
3. The pulse rate is usually accelerated to 140-200 beats per minute. The high rate monitor alarm will be triggered by the onset of ventricular tachycardia.
4. On many occasions, ventricular tachycardia occurs in short runs, or bursts, and then stops spontaneously within a few seconds or so; symptoms may not be impressive in this circumstance.

DANGER IN ACUTE MYOCARDIAL INFARCTION

1. If ventricular tachycardia is sustained and becomes an established rhythm (rather than terminating spontaneously within seconds) the rapid ventricular rate can be expected to produce adverse hemodynamic effects. These are manifested by signs of decreased cardiac output in the form of congestive failure, cardiogenic shock, or cerebral insufficiency. Sudden death may occur during ventricular tachycardia.
2. At any time during the course of ventricular tachycardia, the arrhythmia may *abruptly* change into ventricular fibrillation. For this reason, ventricular tachycardia must be considered in the same life-threatening category as ventricular fibrillation.
3. *RISK:* Extreme danger: an absolute emergency.

TREATMENT

1. About 50 per cent of all episodes of ventricular tachycardia end as abruptly as they began, even without treatment. The transiency of these attacks should not afford comfort since there is a high risk of further episodes of ventricular tachycardia or of the sudden onset of ventricular fibrillation. Even if ventricular tachycardia is of brief duration and stops spontaneously, vigorous antiarrhythmic therapy is nevertheless indicated.

   In this latter circumstance, an infusion containing 1,000 mg of lidocaine in 250 cc of glucose solution should be started promptly to prevent recurrence of this serious arrhythmia. the flow should be set initially at 1 mg (10 microdrops) per minute and adjusted subsequently to control premature beats.

TREATMENT (continued)

2. If ventricular tachycardia is *not* self-limited, and continues, lidocaine should be administered as a rapid injection intravenously in a dosage of 100 mg. After the arrhythmia is controlled with this "push dose", further amounts of lidocaine should be given according to the regimen described in the previous paragraph.

3. Failure to convert ventricular tachycardia to normal sinus rhythm with lidocaine should be considered indication for *immediate, elective precordial shock.* Additional attempts with drug therapy are ill-advised and, as a general rule, if ventricular tachycardia persists by the time the "push dose" of lidocaine is completed, the next step should be cardioversion.

4. Procainamide is probably as effective as lidocaine in terminating ventricular tachycardia and can be used in this situation. Other antiarrhythmic agents are seldom valuable.

5. If ventricular tachycardia recurs despite a continuous infusion of lidocaine or procainamide, hypokalemia should be suspected and an intravenous infusion containing 60 meq of KCL in 1,000 cc glucose solution can be given, even empirically.

6. If, for any reason, ventricular tachycardia persists for five minutes or longer, lactic acidosis may develop and sodium bicarbonate should be given to combat this problem.

NURSING ROLE

1. When the high rate alarm sounds, observe the oscilloscope immediately to identify the cause of this rapid-rate arrhythmia. If ventricular tachycardia is present, an emergency situation exists and the planned program of treatment must be instituted at once.

2. Go to the bedside and examine the patient. If he is *unconscious,* proceed immediately with precordial shock (see Chapter 15). If the patient is *conscious,* assess his clinical state, including the presence of dyspnea and chest pain.

3. Call the physician *at once.*

4. Prepare a syringe containing 100 mg of lidocaine. The physician may instruct the nurse to administer this drug intravenously.

5. Prepare an infusion containing 1,000 mg of lidocaine in 250 cc of glucose solution for use after the "push dose" described above.

6. Allow the write out system of the monitor, or the electrocardiograph, to run continuously until the arrhythmia is terminated.

7. Bring the defibrillator to the bedside and prepare for precordial shock.

8. *Remember that ventricular fibrillation may develop at any time during the course of ventricular tachycardia.*

CASE HISTORY

A 47-year-old-man with an acute myocardial infarction was admitted to the CCU in no distress. Just after the monitor electrodes had been attached and an intravenous infusion of dextrose solution started, the high rate alarm sounded. The nurse recognized immediately that ventricular tachycardia had developed. She examined the patient who complained of the recurrence of chest pain. In accordance with the standing orders of the unit the nurse prepared a syringe containing 50 mg of lidocaine which she injected rapidly into the existing intravenous line. The ventricular tachycardia stopped within 30 seconds. The physician was notified of this event and instructions were given regarding a continuous lidocaine infusion.

VENTRICULAR TACHYCARDIA – IDENTIFYING ECG FEATURES

1. **Rate:**   Usually between 140-200 beats a minute.
2. **P waves:**   Usually buried within the QRS complex and seldom can be identified.
3. **QRS:**   Wide, slurred complexes typical of repetitive premature ventricular contractions.
4. **Conduction:** The ventricles are directly stimulated by an ectopic focus within their walls and beat independently of the atria.
5. **Rhythm:**   The ventricular rhythm is essentially regular.

EXAMPLE: **Sustained Ventricular Tachycardia**

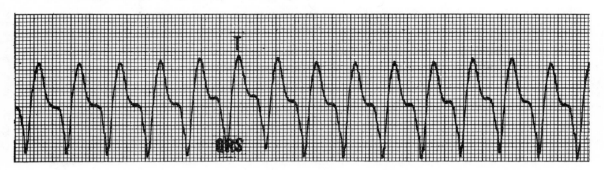

INTERPRETATION OF ECG

Rate: 150 per minute.
P waves: Not identified.
QRS: Widened with bizarre configuration.
Conduction: The impulse arises from a single focus within the ventricle.
Rhythm: Nearly regular.
Comments: The T waves are oppositely directed from the QRS complex characteristic of premature ventricular contractions.

EXAMPLE: **Ventricular Tachycardia Terminating Spontaneously**

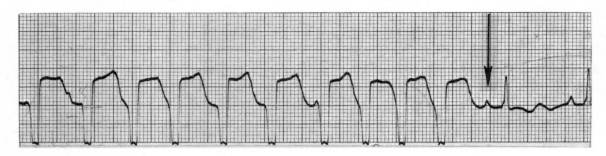

INTERPRETATION OF ECG

Rate: 150 per minute.
P waves: Not identified.
QRS: Widened, slurred and inverted.
Conduction: A series of premature ventricular contractions comprise the rhythm.
Rhythm: Almost regular.
Comments: This episode of ventricular tachycardia stopped spontaneously and was followed by normal sinus rhythm (see arrow). Short runs of this type are the most common form of ventricular tachycardia.

EXAMPLE: **Rapid Ventricular Tachycardia**

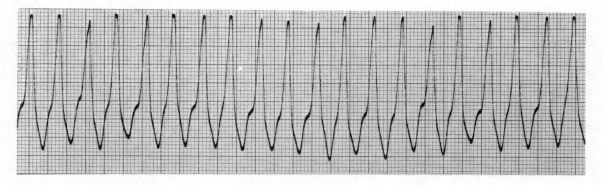

INTERPRETATION OF ECG

Rate:	200 per minute.
P waves:	Not identified.
QRS:	The complexes are widened and notched.
Conduction:	While the ventricles are stimulated from an ectopic focus at a rate of 200 per minute, the atria continued to beat regularly at a slower rate entirely independent of the ventricles.
Rhythm:	Slightly irregular.
Comments:	This very rapid ventricular rate is extremely detrimental to the pumping efficiency of the heart and cannot be tolerated for long periods.

EXAMPLE: **Extreme Ventricular Tachycardia (Ventricular Flutter)**

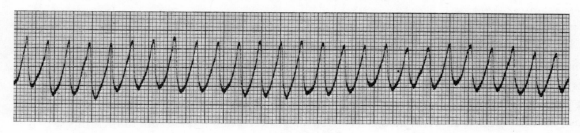

INTERPRETATION OF ECG

Rate:	270 per minute.
P waves:	Not visible.
QRS:	The complexes resemble a helix (similar to a stretched, coiled spring) and occur regularly.
Conduction:	A persistent irritable focus in the ventricle serves as the pacemaker and supersedes the supraventricular centers.
Rhythm:	Almost regular but the interval between the complexes shows slight variation.
Comments:	This extreme form of ventricular tachycardia is sometimes designated as *ventricular flutter*. In many instances it immediately precedes ventricular fibrillation and must be treated with the same urgency as ventricular fibrillation.

BUNDLE BRANCH BLOCK

ETIOLOGY

This arrhythmia is characterized by a *conduction* defect within the ventricular pathway at the level of the right or left branches of the Bundle of His. The cardiac impulse originates normally in the SA node and passes through the AV node to the Bundle of His without difficulty. The impulse is then obstructed in either of the bundle branches because of tissue damage; a left or right bundle branch block then exists. The uninjured branch conducts normally to its ventricle. The affected ventricle is finally activated by impulses which reach it through the interventricular septum from the normally activated side. The time for complete ventricular stimulation is therefore delayed (causing a widened QRS complex).

Bundle branch block may develop acutely as the result of myocardial infarction, but more often, bundle branch block is a consequence of chronic degenerative or fibrotic scarring of the bundle branches. These latter changes antedate the myocardial infarction.

CLINICAL FEATURES

1. Bundle branch block causes no specific symptoms.
2. There are no definite physical findings diagnostic of bundle branch block.
3. While left and right bundle branch blocks produce characteristic patterns and can be readily distinguished from each other electrocardiographically, the single monitor lead is insufficient for this purpose, and a 12 lead ECG is necessary to localize the block.

DANGER IN ACUTE MYOCARDIAL INFARCTION

1. Because bundle branch block does not affect circulatory efficiency, nor specifically warn of impending lethal arrhythmias, this conduction defect is not dangerous in itself. However, the underlying damage to the interventricular septum (which produced the block) has adverse prognostic implications. This poor outlook is particularly apparent with left bundle branch blocks.
2. *Left* bundle branch block obscures the electrocardiographic patterns characteristic of acute myocardial infarction and the diagnosis of infarction becomes difficult.
3. Bundle branch block, either right or left, which develops *acutely* as a result of myocardial infarction, is sometimes transient and may disappear as healing progresses.
4. *RISK:* While not of immediate concern as either a hemodynamic or arrhythmic threat, bundle branch block, nevertheless, may indicate a poor prognosis because of involvement of the interventricular septal area.

TREATMENT

1. There is no specific drug therapy for bundle branch block.
2. On *rare* occasions, bundle branch block may reflect overdosage of digitalis or antiarrhythmic agents (particularly quinidine). In this circumstance, the block may disappear after withdrawal of the drug.
3. The use of transvenous cardiac pacing has been suggested when left bundle branch block exists but the value of this technique is still not proven.

NURSING ROLE

1. If bundle branch block develops *acutely,* identify this conduction defect and document the arrhythmia with an ECG strip.
2. Notify the physician of the sudden occurrence of bundle branch block since this development may indicate spread of the infarction. A 12-lead ECG should be made at this time to localize the site of the block.
3. Careful and frequent clinical observation is particularly important in view of poor prognostic implication of conduction defects.
4. If the patient develops bundle branch block while receiving antiarrhythmic agents, the problem should be discussed with the physician before the next dose is administered.

BUNDLE BRANCH BLOCK — IDENTIFYING ECG FEATURES

1. **Rate:**   Usually normal but bundle branch is not related to rate.
2. **P waves:**   Normal.
3. **QRS:**   *Always* widened to .12 seconds or greater and the configuration of the complex is distorted.
4. **Conduction:** Conduction is normal from the SA node to the site of the block in the left or right bundle branch. The uninvolved bundle then conducts the impulse from the AV node to the Purkinje fibers of the ventricle it supplies. This impulse finally stimulates the blocked side by passing through the interventricular septum. The latter delay causes wide or notched QRS complexes.
5. **Rhythm:**   Regular.

EXAMPLE: **Bundle Branch Block**

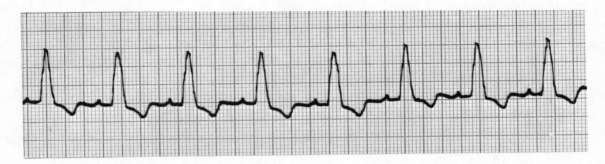

INTERPRETATION OF ECG

Rate: About 80 per minute.

P waves: Normal.

QRS: The contour of the complex is distorted and its duration is 0.14 seconds.

Conduction: The abnormally widened QRS complex (greater than 0.12 seconds) indicates that the time for *total* ventricular activation is prolonged. The impulse, originating in the SA node, is conducted normally until it reaches the bundle branches where transmission is then interrupted in one or the other branch. (See comments).

Rhythm: Regular.

Comments: With a single monitor lead it is usually not possible to distinguish which of the two bundle branches is blocked. This localization, which has prognostic importance, is made with a 12 lead electrocardiogram, from which the respective patterns can be readily identified. The monitor lead indicates only that a conduction defect exists.

CASE HISTORY

A 70-year-old woman was admitted to the CCU with a history of severe substernal pain of 2 hours duration. The nurse noted a widened QRS complex on the initial rhythm strip. A 12-lead ECG was characteristic of a left bundle branch block. Because of this conduction disturbance pattern the diagnosis of acute myocardial infarction could not be made definitely at the time. Despite this uncertainty in diagnosis, the patient was treated as if an acute infarction existed. The question was resolved three days later when the enzyme studies confirmed the presence of acute myocardial infarction.

CHAPTER 14

The Death-Producing Arrhythmias

VENTRICULAR FIBRILLATION
VENTRICULAR STANDSTILL

By contrast, all other arrhythmias are trivial when compared to ventricular fibrillation or ventricular standstill. Both of these arrhythmias are immediate cause of death. They most often develop as a progression of earlier, lesser arrhythmias but occasionally originate *de novo* in a sudden, unexpected fashion. The only hope for survival with either of these lethal arrhythmias is the instant termination of the arrhythmia or the application of resuscitative techniques.

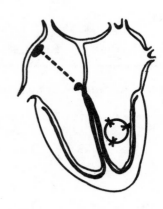

Once ventricular fibrillation or ventricular standstill is detected, a planned treatment program must be started instantly to resuscitate the 'dead' patient*.

Within the coronary care unit the program for resuscitation is distinctly different from that usually administered elsewhere in the hospital. *In the specialized unit the first step in resuscitation is to terminate the arrhythmia.* This means that closed chest massage, ventilation, oxygen, airways and the other procedures normally used at this point are bypassed and the original effort is directed only at treating the *cause* of the catastrophe. It is sometimes difficult for nurses and physicians to realize that there is little reason to start closed chest massage or give oxygen if the catastrophe occurs in the coronary care unit. These techniques are only *interim* measures used to sustain the circulation until definitive action can be taken against the arrhythmia. In the coronary unit everything is in readiness to treat the arrhythmia and therefore these other measures have little importance and, in fact, do no more than waste time. *When ventricular fibrillation occurs in a patient within the unit, external precordial shock must be given as soon as possible by the first person reaching the bedside and should precede any other step!* With ventricular standstill a pacemaker should be used as the fundamental means for resuscitation. While this reversal of the

---

* The older definition of death, namely the absence of the heart beat and peripheral pulses and respiration is obviously inadequate at the present time, since many patients have been restored to useful life despite these signs of circulatory arrest. A more meaningful definition of death must include irreversible damage to brain tissue as the ultimate denominator of death. The need for more precise criteria of death is essential particularly since the advent of heart and organ transplantation.

customary order of treatment is basic to the concept of intensive coronary care, it in no way minimizes the value of closed chest resuscitation as a life-saving measure. The ability to sustain an adequate circulation by means of this latter method has been of inestimable help in combating sudden death. Its greatest usefulness is in sustaining patients until they can be brought to the coronary unit from their home or elsewhere in the hospital. All medical and paramedical personnel should be able to perform closed chest resuscitation.

Once the fatal arrhythmia has been terminated with either precordial shock or cardiac pacing and the circulation has been restored, the remaining program for resuscitation involves the correction of lactic acidosis (which inevitably develops during this brief period) and the subsequent use of drugs to preserve the normal rhythm and prevent further catastrophic episodes. The importance of combating acidosis is mandatory, and large amounts of intravenous bicarbonate solution must be used for this purpose.

VENTRICULAR FIBRILLATION

ETIOLOGY

The individual muscle fibers which jointly comprise the ventricular wall are normally stimulated simultaneously and contract in unison. The fibers then recover together and rest until the next impulse causes another contraction. In ventricular fibrillation an *extraordinary* electrical force arising within the ventricle *repeatedly* stimulates these muscles at a rate so extremely rapid that the recovery period disappears and the individual muscle fibers merely twitch continuously but do not contract. Since the muscular twitching (ventricular fibrillation) is completely ineffective in propelling blood from the ventricles, the circulation stops abruptly, and *death follows within minutes.* Immediately after the onset of ventricular fibrillation, the patient becomes unconscious (and convulsions frequently occur) because of inadequate cerebral oxygenation.

The exact mechanism which triggers ventricular fibrillation is not known with certainty. It would seem that this lethal arrhythmia seldom develops spontaneously and that there is evidence of myocardial irritability in the form of PVC^s prior to the onset of this catastrophic event. It is generally believed that following myocardial infarction the injured myocardium is sensitized so that an abnormal electrical force can initiate chaotic electrical activity (ventricular fibrillation). The usual electrical stimulus responsible for this chain reaction appears to be a premature ventricular contraction which strikes during the vulnerable phase of the cardiac cycle (at the time of the T wave). Electrical forces other than PVC^s also can produce this same lethal effect.

Ventricular fibrillation can develop among patients who have no obvious complications at the time. This form of ventricular fibrillation is defined as *primary ventricular fibrillation.* In contrast, if this lethal arrhythmia occurs among patients dying of advanced left ventricular failure as a terminal rhythm, it is classified as *secondary ventricular fibrillation.* This distinction is very important because death can be predictably *prevented* by prompt defibrillation in all instances of *primary* ventricular fibrillation, while the *secondary* form is seldom responsive to resuscitation because of the underlying heart failure.

CLINICAL FEATURES

1. The patient loses consciousness almost instantly after the onset of ventricular fibrillation. It is safe to assume that a *conscious* patient does not have ventricular fibrillation.
2. The peripheral pulses cannot be detected and there are no heart sounds audible; the blood pressure is unobtainable.
3. The pupils dilate rapidly and convulsions may occur as a result of immediate cerebral anoxia.
4. Cyanosis develops quickly and *total cessation of circulation is evident.*

DANGER IN ACUTE MYOCARDIAL INFARCTION

1. *Death occurs within minutes after the onset of ventricular fibrillation unless the arrhythmia is terminated.* The exact duration of life with primary ventricular fibrillation depends on several factors—the most important of which probably is the patient's age. For example, an 80-year-old man may die in less than a minute while a much younger patient may survive 3 or more minutes before death is irreversible. For this reason, a precise time cannot be defined for successful resuscitation. An average time is probably *2 minutes.*
2. Although ventricular fibrillation can still be terminated after this critical 2-minute period, irreversible brain damage may have developed.
3. *RISK: SUPREME DANGER! Death is inevitable unless resuscitation is accomplished immediately.*

VENTRICULAR FIBRILLATION

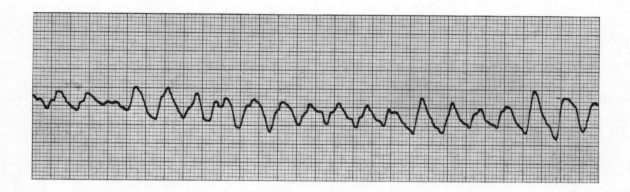

TREATMENT

The treatment program for *primary* ventricular fibrillation can be considered as four phases:

1. *Recognition*

    The initial step in the treatment of ventricular fibrillation is immediate identification of the arrhythmia. When ventricular fibrillation occurs, the alarm system of the monitor is triggered. The electrocardiographic pattern of ventricular fibrillation is readily distinguished by a series of chaotic waves which have no uniformity and are bizarre in their configuration. If the pattern cannot be identified instantly, no further time should be dedicated to monitor observation. Instead, the observer should proceed immediately to the bedside and ascertain if the patient is unconscious as the result of circulatory arrest.

    If the patient is *unconscious* and peripheral pulses are not detectable, the planned treatment program should be initiated instantly.

2. *Termination of ventricular fibrillation*

    Precordial shock (defibrillation) is the first and only treatment for ventricular fibrillation. *This shock should be administered by the first person to reach the bedside, whether a nurse or physician.* Defibrillation must be accomplished within 2 minutes; the sooner the shock is delivered, the greater the chance for recovery.

    It is essential to realize that precordial shock must always be the *initial* step in treatment, and that time should never be wasted with customary cardiopulmonary resuscitation techniques.

    Regardless of the machine used to perform defibrillation, the maximal energy setting (400 watt seconds) should always be used.

3. *Correction of lactic acidosis*

    Every patient who develops ventricular fibrillation can be expected to have lactic acidosis as a result of the cessation of circulation regardless of the brevity of the circulatory arrest. (The etiology of this problem has been discussed in the section on cardiogenic shock).

    Sodium bicarbonate should, therefore, be administered intravenously immediately after the arrhythmia is terminated.

4. *Prevention of recurrence of ventricular fibrillation*

    The myocardial irritability, which led to ventricular fibrillation in the first place, represents a potential threat for subsequent episodes. In other words, the source of the original problem still persists and must be treated vigorously if further episodes of this lethal arrhythmia are to be prevented. This prevention is best accomplished by the use of a continuous infusion of lidocaine (1,000 mg in 500 cc of glucose) at a rate designed to control or at least minimize premature ventricular contractions.

174

VENTRICULAR FIBRILLATION — IDENTIFYING ECG FEATURES

The ECG pattern is characterized by a rapid, repetitive series of *chaotic* waves originating in the ventricles that have no uniformity and are bizarre in configuration. PQRST waves cannot specifically be identified. The complexes differ from each other and occur in completely irregular fashion. A typical example of ventricular fibrillation is shown below.

This gross irregularity can hardly be mistaken for any other arrhythmia. The only other possibility to account for such gross distortion is a disorder of the monitor or the electrocardiograph machine.

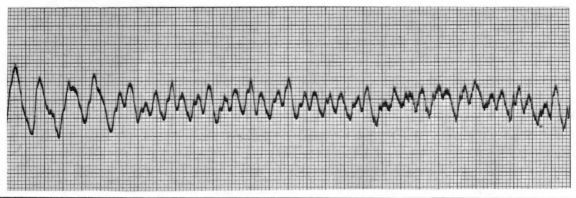

CASE HISTORY

Note: The following case history describes the first instance of life saving defibrillation performed by a nurse in the absence of a physician. This event took place in 1963 and became the precedent for the now common practice of defibrillation by nurses.

A 72-year-old male was admitted to the Coronary Care Unit with a history of chest pain that had subsided by the time of his arrival. He had no complaints; in fact, he wanted to go home. An electrocardiogram showed an acute myocardial infarction. Physical examination was normal and there was no evidence of complications. He remained in normal sinus rhythm with a rate ranging from 60 to 74 beats per minute. Occasional premature beats were noted.

Some 60 hours after admission, in the middle of the night, the monitor alarm sounded. The nurse instantly recognized ventricular fibrillation on the oscilloscope and ran to the bedside where the patient was found to be unconscious. She immediately called the physician and set a timing device for 2 minutes. She turned on the defibrillator, set the energy level at 400 watt-seconds, and applied electrode paste to the defibrillator paddles. The two minute interval timer sounded before the physician had arrived. (The practice at that time was for the nurse to proceed with defibrillation herself only if a physician had not arrived within two minutes.) The nurse then defibrillated the patient without further delay. Normal sinus rhythm was established almost immediately (see recording below.) The patient survived and is still alive six years later.

EXAMPLE:

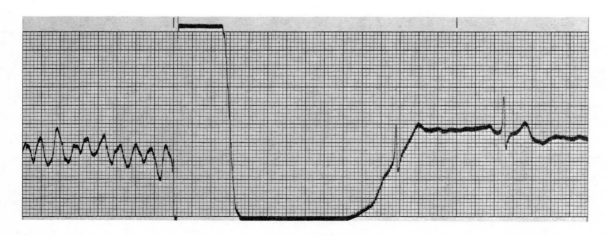

NURSING ROLE

1. Ventricular fibrillation will trigger the alarm system of the monitor. (Either the high or low rate alarm may sound.)

2. Identify the bizarre irregular pattern of ventricular fibrillation. Even if in doubt, do not waste time with further monitor observation. Allow the electrocardiographic record to run continuously.

3. Go to the bedside and examine the patient. If he is conscious, and responds to your call, ventricular fibrillation is *not* the problem. If the patient *is unconscious,* ascertain the absence of peripheral pulses and heart sounds.

4. If assistance is available, ask that the emergency system call be sounded and that an automatic timer be activated.

5. Turn on the power switch of the defibrillator and set the instrument dial at the maximum energy (400 watt-seconds). If a DC defibrillator is used, make certain the synchronizer switch is in the "OFF" position.

6. *Perform defibrillation immediately. Specifically, do not wait for the arrival of a physician or other nursing personnel before proceeding.*

    Steps in defibrillation:

    a. Make certain the machine is *on;* that the energy level is maximum; and that the synchronizer is *"off."*

    b. Apply a generous amount of electrode paste to the defibrillator paddles and spread the jelly evenly by approximating the surfaces of the paddles.

    c. Hold the paddles *tightly* against the chest wall. The exact position of the paddles is not important as long as the current will traverse the heart.

    d. Trigger the discharge mechanism of the defibrillator.

    Remember that survival after ventricular fibrillation is directly dependent on the rapidity with which the shock is delivered.

7. Immediately after the shock has been delivered, observe the monitor to see if the fibrillation has terminated. (If an oscilloscope is not visible from the bedside, the prompt return of peripheral pulses or the return of consciousness reflects successful defibrillation.)

8. If ventricular fibrillation persists despite the initial attempt, a second or third shock should be given promptly.

9. If defibrillation has not been effective at this point, (a very unlikely situation with proper technique), additional shocks are probably unwarranted at this time. External cardiac massage and mouth-to-mouth resuscitation, should be started without delay. A rapid injection of sodium bicarbonate (40 mEq.) must be administered during this period, after which defibrillation should be attempted again.

10. Unsuccessful defibrillation after these measures usually implies that ventricular fibrillation is *secondary* to advanced left ventricular failure. Survival in this circumstance is unlikely.

EXAMPLE: **The onset of Ventricular Fibrillation**

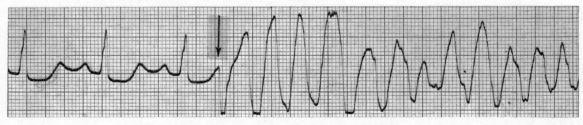

Comments: A premature ventricular contraction striking the T wave of the preceding complex (see arrow) precipitates ventricular fibrillation.

VENTRICULAR STANDSTILL

ETIOLOGY

If the electrical stimulus to the ventricles becomes inadequate or ceases entirely, the ventricles will not contract effectively; this state is designated as *ventricular standstill**. The end result of this catastrophe is the same as with ventricular fibrillation, namely, sudden death.

Ventricular standstill may develop in two ways: (1) as a primary arrhythmia *(primary ventricular standstill)* or, (2) as a terminal arrhythmia during far advanced left ventricular failure *(secondary ventricular standstill)*.

In *primary* ventricular standstill *atrial* impulses continue to be discharged normally but are blocked or dissipated before reaching the ventricle. While this event often occurs with seeming suddenness, in fact, previous evidence of heart block usually precedes the onset of this type of ventricular standstill. When ventricular contractions either stop or become too slow to maintain effective circulation, unconsciousness develops and *death occurs*. However, on some occasions ventricular standstill is only *transient* and conduction and stimulation spontaneously return. Such *intermittent* episodes are characterized by syncope and are described as *Stokes-Adams attacks.*

Secondary ventricular standstill is the ultimate cause of death among many patients with cardiogenic shock or heart failure. The poor tissue perfusion associated with such heart failure produces anoxemia and electrolyte imbalances which depress electrical conductivity. At a critical point, the electrical activity becomes insufficient to stimulate contraction and ventricular standstill develops. This *secondary* type of standstill seldom responds to resuscitative techniques, including pacing, because of the continuation of the basic circulatory problem that caused the arrhythmia originally. Death from secondary ventricular standstill may occur gradually and electrical activity may continue while muscle contractions become weak and ineffective in propelling blood from the ventricles. This condition is designated as mechanical, or "power" failure, in contrast to failure of electrical stimulation and conduction.

CLINICAL FEATURES

1. At the bedside, ventricular standstill *cannot* be distinguished from ventricular fibrillation. In both instances there is complete cessation of circulation. No heart beat can be heard; the blood pressure is unobtainable; signs of cerebral anoxia (unconsciousness, dilated pupils) develop. *Death follows within minutes.*
2. Ventricular standstill can be recognized on the electrocardiogram and clearly differentiated from ventricular fibrillation. It is obviously necessary to ascertain which of these arrhythmias is present because of the totally different therapies employed in resuscitation.

DANGER IN ACUTE MYOCARDIAL INFARCTION

1. *Primary* ventricular standstill is an *immediate* and direct cause of death unless resuscitation can be accomplished within a minute or two. This catastrophic arrhythmia is less common than primary ventricular fibrillation.
2. *Secondary* ventricular standstill is almost inevitably fatal with current means of therapy.
3. *RISK: Ventricular standstill is undoubtedly the most dreaded and dangerous of all arrhythmias.* Even with primary ventricular standstill, the results with resuscitation are distressingly poor (and certainly less successful than resuscitation from ventricular fibrillation).

*There is some confusion regarding the proper terminology of this catastrophe. The terms "ventricular standstill," "ventricular asystole," "cardiac standstill," and "cardiac arrest" are used interchangeably to designate cessation of heart action.

At the bedside, without an electrocardiogram, one cannot distinguish ventricular standstill from ventricular fibrillation since both arrhythmias are characterized by the absence of audible heart sounds. In this situation, it is common practice to classify cessation of the circulation as *cardiac arrest* even though ventricular fibrillation may actually be at fault.

In the coronary care unit, where the lethal arrhythmia can be specifically identified, it is poor practice to use the general term "cardiac arrest" when the arrhythmia is actually ventricular standstill or ventricular fibrillation.

VENTRICULAR STANDSTILL

TREATMENT
The treatment program has 4 phases:

1. *Recognition*

   When primary ventricular standstill occurs, the low rate alarm of the monitor system is activated. The electrocardiographic pattern of ventricular standstill is identified by the *absence* of the ventricular (QRS) complex, while atrial activity (P waves) continues. As with ventricular fibrillation, if the ECG pattern cannot be recognized instantly, no further time should be spent in attempting to clarify the diagnosis. The observer should examine the patient immediately and ascertain if the patient is unconscious.

2. *Termination of ventricular standstill*

   (a) As noted previously, ventricular standstill is usually preceded by evidence of advanced heart block or extreme bradycardia. Thus the arrhythmia cannot truly be considered as unexpected; only the onset is sudden. On the basis of these warnings most patients should have had a transvenous pacing catheter inserted before ventricular standstill ever developed.

   If a *demand* pacemaker was inserted prophylactically, the pacemaker will function at the onset of ventricular standstill and the arrhythmia will be terminated instantly. If a *set rate* pacemaker was inserted on a standby basis, the instrument must be manually activated within 30 to 60 seconds to restore the heart beat.

   (b) If primary ventricular standstill develops *before* a transvenous pacing catheter has been inserted (because of abrupt onset or failure to heed the warning of previous heart block), *external* pacing can be attempted. This latter technique is *much less* successful than transvenous pacing.

   (c) A more effective method for pacing the heart in the absence of an indwelling transvenous pacemaker involves the use of a wire electrode inserted directly into the myocardium through the chest wall. This technique, called transthoracic pacing, is described in Chapter 15.

   (d) In the event that immediate pacing cannot be accomplished with any of the previous techniques, no additional time should be wasted and the usual program of cardiopulmonary resuscitation should be started instantly.

   (e) Intracardiac injection of epinephrine is occasionally successful in restoring the heart beat, but this therapy should not be used prior to pacing attempts and/or cardiopulmonary resuscitation.

3. *Correction of lactic acidosis*

   Lactic acidosis should be anticipated in every patient who sustains ventricular standstill, and sodium bicarbonate should be administered intravenously as soon as possible. Unless this acidosis is corrected, pacing is likely to be ineffective and ventricular standstill will recur.

4. *Prevention Recurrence*

   Every patient who survives ventricular standstill should be paced thereafter until there is no evidence of heart block remaining. The transvenous pacemaker should then be left in place on a standby basis for at least one more week.

VENTRICULAR STANDSTILL

NURSING ROLE

1. *If a transvenous standby pacemaker IS in place when primary ventricular standstill occurs.*

   a. When the low rate alarm sounds, attempt to identify the electrocardiographic pattern. Go to the bedside at once and observe the patient. If the patient is awake and converses, it is quite certain that a false alarm has occurred.

   b. If the patient is *not* conscious, and has no peripheral pulses or heart sounds, the pacemaker should be turned on instantly. (If the pacemaker, either set rate or demand, was already functioning, primary ventricular standstill would not have occurred.)

   c. The success of pacing will be evident by the prompt return of consciousness and the presence of peripheral pulses.

   d. Sound the emergency alarm for the physician on call.

   e. If for any reason pacing is *not* effective in restoring circulation, external cardiac massage and mouth-to-mouth resuscitation should be started by the nurse without delay.

2. *If a standby transvenous pacemaker is NOT in place when ventricular standstill occurs.*

   a. Proceed to the bedside immediately after the low rate alarm has sounded and verify the clinical state of the patient.

   b. Sound the emergency alarm system.

   c. Deliver a sharp blow to the chest wall directly over the heart. This simple procedure may sometimes re-establish the heart beat and is always worth trying.

   d. If *external* pacing electrodes are in place, or can be attached within seconds, this type of pacing should be started. Turn on the power switch of the external pacemaker as soon as possible. *Do not wait for the physician.*

   e. If the heart beat has not been restored within 1 minute after the onset of external pacing, there is little likelihood of success in the future and such pacing should be discontinued.

   f. Begin external cardiac massage and mouth-to-mouth breathing; continue this resuscitative attempt until assistance arrives.

   g. Transthoracic pacing equipment should be brought to bedside for immediate use by the physician.

   h. An assistant should prepare a syringe containing 40 mEq. of sodium bicarbonate solution for immediate intravenous injection. A subsequent infusion containing 400 mEq. of sodium bicarbonate should be available.

   i. In the event of failure with other measures, the physician may inject 1 cc of 1:1000 epinephrine directly into the heart. Prepare a syringe with an intracardiac needle for this purpose.

CASE HISTORY

A 71-year-old man was admitted to the CCU with obvious signs of advanced left ventricular failure. The electrocardiogram revealed an anteroseptal myocardial infarction and a rhythm strip showed sinus tachycardia with a rate of 132 per minute. He was treated with digitalis, ethacrynic acid and oxygen. The response to therapy was poor and the patient continued with marked dyspnea. During the course of treatment the heart rate slowed rather abruptly to 58 and a nodal rhythm was recognized on the ECG. A transvenous pacemaker was inserted but pacing was ineffective and 5 minutes later the patient suddenly lost consciousness. The nurse was unable to record a blood pressure and no peripheral pulses were palpable. The monitor showed isolated, broad, distorted ventricular complexes occurring about 15-20 times a minute. Resuscitation attempts were unsuccessful. The cause of death was advanced left ventricular failure. The terminal rhythm was secondary ventricular standstill.

PRIMARY VENTRICULAR STANDSTILL
IDENTIFYING ECG FEATURES

1. **Rate:** At the onset of ventricular standstill the ventricles cease to contract.
2. **P waves:** The P waves are usually normal and continue for a period of time despite the cessation of ventricular complexes.
3. **QRS:** Absent.
4. **Conduction:** Atrial activity continues but there is no conduction to the ventricles which cease to function.
5. **Rhythm:** There is no heart beat once the ventricles stop.

EXAMPLE: **Primary Ventricular Standstill**

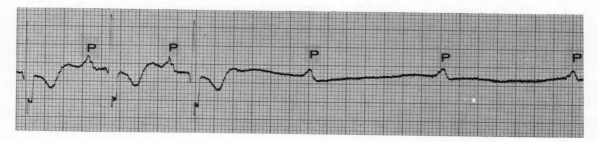

INTERPRETATION OF ECG

Rate: After the third QRS complex, the ventricles ceased to contract and there is no heart rate.

P waves: Atrial activity (P waves) continue after ventricular standstill.

QRS: Absent when ventricular standstill occurs.

Conduction: The ventricles are not stimulated and do not contract. Atrial activity exists independently but the impulse is not transmitted to the ventricles.

Rhythm: Total cessation of ventricular activity.

Comments: The sudden onset of ventricular standstill developed in the presence of first degree heart block in this instance. Ventricular standstill more commonly occurs during complete heart block as shown in the following example.

EXAMPLE: **Ventricular Standstill Developing During Complete Heart Block.**

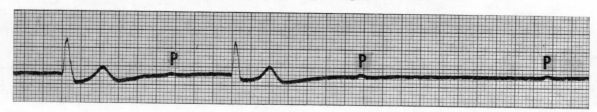

SECONDARY VENTRICULAR STANDSTILL
IDENTIFYING ECG FEATURES

1. **Rate:** Electrical activity in the ventricles may continue producing infrequent QRS complexes (rate 10 - 30 per minute)
2. **P waves:** Absent since atrial death has occurred.
3. **QRS:** Wide slurred complexes at a very slow rate.
4. **Conduction:** There is no conduction through the heart and the stimulus is of ventricular origin.
5. **Rhythm:** Although the QRS complexes may occur at regular intervals there is no effective ventricular pumping function and therefore no peripheral pulses.

EXAMPLE: **Secondary Ventricular Standstill**

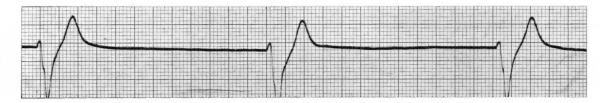

INTERPRETATION OF ECG

Rate: Less than 30 per minute.
P wave: Not present.
QRS: Very wide and distorted.
Conduction: The isolated complexes arise in the ventricle and there is no conduction through the heart.
Rhythm: The occasional ventricular complexes do not actually constitute a cardiac rhythm. They represent isolated electrical activity but are not associated with effective ventricular contractions.
Comments: Cardiac pacing is seldom effective in secondary ventricular standstill. The myocardium is unable to respond to the electrical stimulus because of advanced ischemia.

EXAMPLE: **Dying Heart**

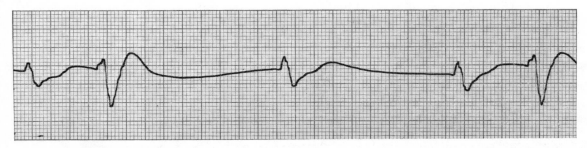

Comments: While there is occasional electrical activity in the ventricle, true stimulation of the myocardium does not occur. The bizarre distorted complexes continued for several minutes even though the patient was clinically dead. This pattern is common among patients dying of advanced left ventricular failure (secondary ventricular standstill).

CHAPTER 15

The Electrical Treatment of Arrhythmias
Cardiac Pacing
Precordial Shock

In previous chapters reference was made on several occasions to the use of cardiac pacing and precordial shock for the treatment of various arrhythmias. Because these electrical methods have been developed in recent years and are unfamiliar to most nurses this subject is considered in greater detail in this chapter.

CARDIAC PACING

If the inherent electrical system of the heart fails, for some reason, it is possible to stimulate the myocardium and induce ventricular contractions with electrical impulses from an external source. This is achieved by the use of a device, called a pacemaker, which discharges repetitive electrical impulses so that an effective heart rate can be maintained and life preserved. These stimuli can be delivered to the heart in three basic ways: 1) by means of an electrode placed on the chest wall (external pacing); 2) by inserting a needle electrode through the chest wall into the myocardium (transthoracic pacing); 3) by passing a small electrode through the venous system into the right ventricular cavity (transvenous pacing). Pacing can also be accomplished with electrodes attached directly to the epicardial surface of the heart. Since this technique (permanent cardiac pacing) requires a thoracotomy it has no application in the treatment of acute myocardial infarction and is reserved for chronic heart block.

External Cardiac Pacing

This method of stimulation, historically the first employed to pace the heart, is now used only as a desperation measure in the emergency treatment of ventricular standstill. The technique has been practically discarded in coronary care programs because of its unpredictable effectiveness. Experience has shown that external pacing is seldom successful in resuscitation from ventricular standstill unless pacing is initiated within 15-30 seconds after asystole develops. Furthermore, the magnitude of electrical current required to effect ventricular contraction through the closed chest wall is so great that the stimulus causes local pain, intense contractions of the skeletal muscles, and (with prolonged use) skin burns. For these reasons external cardiac pacing is unsuitable for the preventative treatment of warning arrhythmias (e.g., second or third degree heart block).

181

182

Despite these obvious disadvantages external cardiac pacing has nonetheless been life-saving in some instances (see Fig. 15-1 demonstrating the restoration of sinus rhythm after primary ventricular standstill) and on this basis the technique is worth noting.

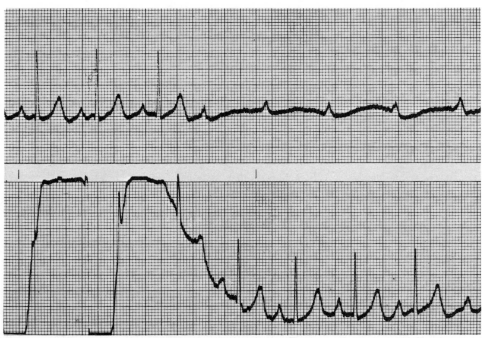

PRIMARY VENTRICULAR STANDSTILL (STOKES — ADAMS ATTACK) SUCCESSFULLY TREATED WITH EXTERNAL PACEMAKER.

Fig. 15-1

Technique of External Pacing

1) A small (1½ inch) metal electrode is attached to the chest wall in the left precordial area and anchored firmly to the skin with adhesive tape. A second electrode (the ground electrode) is placed on the opposite side of the chest or under the tip of the left scapula.

2) The electrode wires are then connected to the pacemaking device. This pulse generator may be a separate instrument or may be part of the monitor system.

3) The energy output dial of the pacemaker should be turned to its *maximum* setting. Lesser energies should not be attempted initially; however, the strength of the impulse can be reduced if the myocardium responds and the patient becomes conscious.

4) The pacing rate is set at 80 impulses per minute.

5) If the heart does not respond to these stimuli within a minute, external pacing should be abandoned and cardiopulmonary resuscitation started instantly.

Transthoracic Pacing

Ventricular stimulation can also be achieved by means of a thin wire electrode inserted directly into the myocardium by way of a needle introduced through the chest wall. This technique, like external cardiac pacing, is used only for emergency resuscitation following primary ventricular standstill. The major advantage of this method is the rapidity with which pacing can be initiated. The necessary equipment consists only of a transthoracic needle and a small length of steel wire which serves as the electrode. Furthermore with the electrode in the myocardium only minimal electrical energy is needed to pace the heart and the stimulus does not produce the pain or violent muscle contractions which accompany external pacing. Any independent, battery powered pacemaker can be used as a power source.

Technique of Transthoracic Pacing

1) A long, 18 gauge, transthoracic needle is introduced through the chest wall, usually in the interspace between the left 5th and 6th ribs (in the precordial area) and advanced superiorly toward the direction of the right shoulder. When the needle encounters the outer cardiac surface it is passed another 5 mm. directly into the ventricular wall.

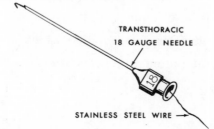

TRANSTHORACIC
18 GAUGE NEEDLE

Fig. 15-2

STAINLESS STEEL WIRE →

2) Once the needle has been placed in this way, a thin, 35 gauge, stainless steel wire (a suture wire is satisfactory) with a tiny hook bent into its end (see Fig. 15-2) is introduced through the needle into the ventricular wall. The needle is then withdrawn, leaving the wire electrode hooked in place.

3) As with all other pacing systems a ground, or indifferent, electrode is required to create a circuit. This involves no more than placing a customary wire suture in the chest wall to serve this purpose.

4) The electrode wire from the myocardium is connected to the *negative* pole of the pacemaker and the indifferent electrode to the *positive* pole.

5) The energy setting of the battery powered pacemaker is adjusted to 10-15 milliamperes and the pacing rate established at 80 per minute.

Transvenous Pacing

The heart can be safely and effectively stimulated from a small electrode placed within the right ventricle. This pacing electrode is introduced into a superficial vein and then advanced through the peripheral venous system, the vena cava, and the right atrium until it is lodged against the endocardial surface of the right ventricle. The electrical stimulus is furnished by a small battery-powered pulse generator. This technique, called *transvenous pacing* is now used routinely in most coronary care units.

The prime reason for transvenous pacing is to *prevent* ventricular standstill. As noted in the previous chapters, ventricular standstill seldom develops spontaneously and, in most instances, this lethal arrhythmia is preceded by second degree and third degree heart block. By pacing the heart when these advanced forms of heart block exist it is possible to avoid ventricular standstill.

In addition to this fundamental indication, transvenous pacing is also employed to treat other bradyarrhythmias. It is now a common practice to increase the heart rate by transvenous pacing when arrhythmias such as sinus bradycardia or nodal rhythm prove refractory to usual drug therapy and compromise the cardiac output.

Pacing is also used to control resistant ectopic rhythms (for example, frequent premature ventricular contractions) which are rate related. By pacing the heart faster than the existing rate, premature beats can often be suppressed. This principle is called *overdriving* the heart.

The Equipment for Transvenous Pacing

There are two components to a transvenous pacing system:

1) A battery operated pulse generator which serves as the source of electrical impulses. Both the rate and the intensity of these impulses can be controlled.

2) A wire catheter which carried the current from the pacemaker to the myocardium. The distal end of the catheter contains one or two small electrodes which make contract with the endocardial surface.

The Pulse Generator

There are two types of pacemakers: set rate and demand. The differences between these pacing devices and their respective functions are considered in the following paragraphs.

Set Rate, Or Fixed, Pulse Generators

This device, the first available for transvenous pacing, is used infrequently today in most coronary care units. Nevertheless, it is important to consider the design and operation of set rate pacemakers to understand the newer pacemakers now in use. Very simply, these battery powered pulse generators initiate impulses at a fixed or set rate. For example, if the rate dial is position at 60 per minute one impulse is fired every second. Each stimulus produces a QRS complex (See Fig. 15-3). The resultant complex is widened and resembles a left bundle branch block pattern. (This is understandable since the electrode delivering the stimulus is in the *right* ventricle and the impulse must be transmitted from this site to the *left* ventricle resulting in a delay in full ventricular activation.)

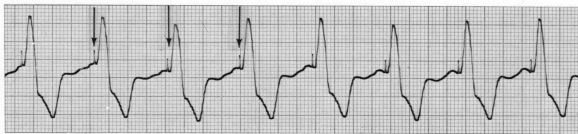

Fig. 15-3

Set rate pacing has one serious drawback: The instrument disregards the existing electrical activity of the heart. Thus, a natural beat from the heart and a pacing stimulus may occur at the same time, as shown in Fig. 15-4. This is called *"competition."*

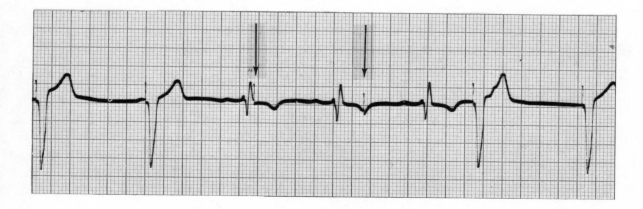

Fig. 15-4

186

When the paced and natural rhythms compete in this way, serious arrhythmias may arise particularly if the pacing stimulus happens to hit the T wave of the preceding beat (usually a premature ventricular contraction). The arrival of the pacing stimulus during this vunerable period (see page 199) may induce repetitive firing in the form of ventricular tachycardia or ventricular fibrillation as shown in Fig. 15-5. While competition

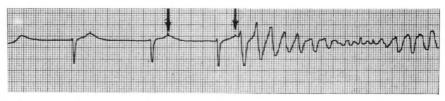

Fig. 15-5

certainly does not result in ventricular arrhythmias in all (or most) instances as apparent in Fig. 15-6 where the pacing stimulus hits the T wave of a premature ventricular contraction

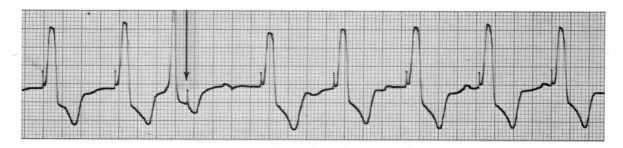

Fig. 15-6

without provoking repetitive firing, this potential threat nevertheless exists. It is for this reason that set rate pacing is undesirable, particularly when the underlying cardiac rhythm is irregular (e.g., complete heart block with frequent PVCs as noted on page 157). This form of pacing should be reserved theoretically for only slow, regular arrhythmias. In the treatment of acute myocardial infarction, where ectopic beats are so common, set rate pacing is less-than-optimal.

The Demand Pulse Generator

To avoid the potential danger of competition associated with fixed rate pacing, a new type of pulse generator was developed. This pacemaker sends an impulse only on *demand* rather than at a fixed rate.

The principle of demand pacing is as follows: the pacemaker fires an impulse *only* if a QRS complex does *not* occur within a preset time interval. If a QRS complex *does* occur in this designated period, the pacemaker withholds the pacing impulse. For this reason, a pacing impulse cannot strike the T wave of a premature ventricular contraction since the pacemaker will recognize this ectopic beat (which occurs within the preset interval) and will not fire an impulse. On the other hand if the pacemaker does *not* sense a natural or ectopic beat it discharges an impulse at a set rate. An example of demand pacing is shown in the Fig. 15-7. Note that the pacemaker stops discharging impulses when a series of normal beats occur (all of which fall within the pre-set time interval). When the interval is again exceeded, the pacemaker begins to discharge.*

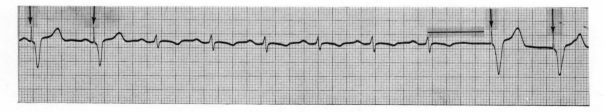

Fig. 15-7

In order for a pacemaker to function on demand it must be given an electrocardiographic signal indicating that a natural or ectopic beat has occurred. This is achieved by having the catheter tip serve as an exploring intracavitary electrode so that each QRS complex is transmitted back to a sensing device within the pacemaker. Thus the catheter serves to relay electrocardiographic signals *to* the pacemaker and pacing impulses *from* the device (see Fig. 15-8).

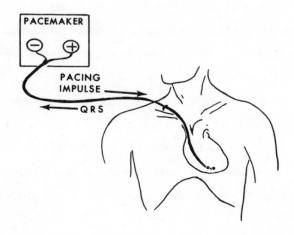

Fig. 15-8

* In addition to this R wave-inhibited device other types of demand pacemakers have been developed. One of these functions by superimposing the pacing impulse directly on the R wave of the natural or ectopic beats. These pacing impulses are ineffective because they arrive when the myocardium is refractory to stimulation. If a QRS complex does not occur within the preset interval the pacemaker then discharges at a set rate.

188

Types of Catheter Electrodes

There are two basic types of catheter electrodes: those with a single electrode incorporated in the tip of the catheter (unipolar electrode) and those with two electrodes about 1cm. apart at the distal end of the catheter (bipolar electrode) as shown in Fig. 15-9. In order to stimulate the heart, the electrical impulse from the pacemaker must flow between two poles (or electrodes) to create an electrical circuit. With the unipolar

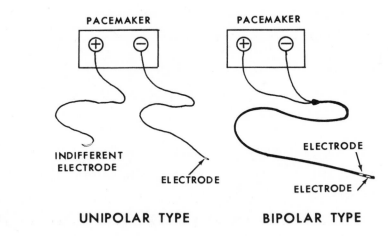

Fig. 15-9   **UNIPOLAR TYPE**   **BIPOLAR TYPE**

catheter only one electrode (the negative pole) is within the heart and it is necessary to establish a second electrode (the positive pole) to complete the circuit. A wire sature placed in the skin of the chest wall serves as this indifferent electrode.

The bipolar catheter electrode obviates the need for a separate skin electrode since both electrodes are incorporated into the catheter itself. Because of this dual electrode system, bipolar catheters are of greater diameter (larger gauge) than unipolar catheters and therefore may be more difficult to pass to the ventricle. Despite this problem bipolar catheters are considered preferable to unipolar types because the presence of two adjacent electrodes within the heart enhances the likelihood of electrode contact with the endocardial surface of the ventricle, a requirement for successful pacing. With a unipolar catheter the electrode may be easily displaced from the ventricular wall and interrupt effective pacing.

Technique of Transvenous Pacing

Catheter Insertion

a) Selection of a vein

The pacing electrode can be introduced into the venous system through either an antecubital vein, a jugular vein, or a subclavian vein. The selection of the vein to be used for this purpose is a matter of individual preference. While an arm vein is usually the easiest to enter percutaneously, the route to the heart is long and tortuous so that advancement of the catheter is often difficult. Furthermore, movement of the arm may displace the catheter once it has been properly positioned. The jugular and subclavian veins, being closer to the superior vena cava are shorter and more direct routes to the ventricle. For this reason, and since displacement of the catheter is less likely, these sites are preferable.

b) Introduction of Catheter Electrode

Once a particular vein is selected, the surrounding skin area must be scrupulously cleaned as for any surgical procedure and draped to prevent contamination.

Several specially designed needles are available for catheter insertion. Most of the placement units consist of a large-bore needle (with a stylus) and a thin plastic sheath which fits over this cannula. After the skin is infiltrated with a local anesthetic, the unit is inserted into the vein; the needle (and stylus) is then removed leaving the plastic sheath positioned in the vein.

The catheter electrode is introduced through this plastic sheath into the vein and advanced to the right ventricle. After the electrode is in proper position within the ventricle, the plastic conduit is removed so that the catheter then extends directly through the skin.

In some instances where needle penetration of the skin or vein is difficult a small surgical "cut-down" incision can be made to facilitate vein entry.

c) Passage of the catheter

Regardless of the site of introduction, the catheter is advanced slowly to the superior vena cava, into the right atrium, through the tricuspid valve and to the right ventricle where it is positioned against the endocardial surface. This pathway of the catheter is shown in Fig. 15-10. Two methods are available to guide the catheter to its ultimate position in the ventricle. The first involves fluoroscopy where the radio-opaque catheter is directly visualized during its passage. Although this technique is very desirable, most coronary care units are not equipped with the expensive apparatus needed for this purpose (i.e., a portable fluoroscope with an image intensifier); therefore, patients have to be moved to either an x-ray department or to a catheterization laboratory when a catheter is to be positioned with this technique. This separation of the patient from the prepared setting of the coronary unit poses obvious risks and is hardly ideal.

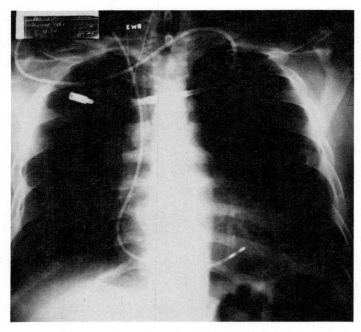

Fig. 15-10

The catheter can also be guided to the right ventricle by electrocardiographic means. This method can be performed in the coronary care unit and avoids the danger of moving the patient. The principle of this "blind" technique is as follows: as the electrode is being advanced to the heart an electrocardiogram can be recorded *through* the catheter by attaching its free end to the chest lead (V lead) terminal of the electrocardiographic machine. In other words, the catheter tip serves as an exploring electrode from within the heart. The resulting tracing is called an *intracavitary* electrocardiogram. Because the ECG patterns from the vena cava, the atrium, and the right ventricle all have different configurations it is possible to identity the position of the electrode in this way. Typical ECG patterns from these various locations are shown in Fig. 15-11. Note the large distinctive complexes recorded when the catheter enters the ventricle.

When this method of electrocardiographic guidance is used it is necessary to connect all of the limb-leads just as if a customary electrocardiogram were to be recorded. The only difference is that the chest (V) lead, rather than being used as a skin electrode, is joined to the free end of the catheter.

Attachment of the Catheter Electrode to the Pacemaking Device

The pacemaker device has two terminals for connection of the electrodes; these are clearly marked as "positive" (+) and "negative" (−). When a unipolar electrode is used the free end of the catheter is attached to the negative (−) terminal of the pacemaker and the wire from the skin electrode (suture) is connected to the positive (+) terminal.

Intracavitary electrocardiograms (5) parts

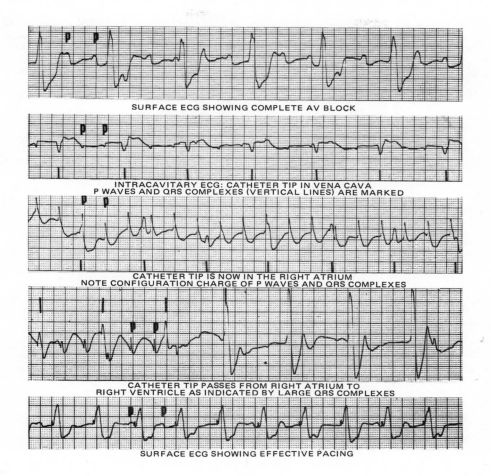

SURFACE ECG SHOWING COMPLETE AV BLOCK

INTRACAVITARY ECG: CATHETER TIP IN VENA CAVA
P WAVES AND QRS COMPLEXES (VERTICAL LINES) ARE MARKED

CATHETER TIP IS NOW IN THE RIGHT ATRIUM
NOTE CONFIGURATION CHARGE OF P WAVES AND QRS COMPLEXES

CATHETER TIP PASSES FROM RIGHT ATRIUM TO
RIGHT VENTRICLE AS INDICATED BY LARGE QRS COMPLEXES

SURFACE ECG SHOWING EFFECTIVE PACING

Fig. 15-11

With a bipolar catheter electrode the two wires extending from the catheter can be connected to the terminals without concern about positive or negative poles.

Rate of Pacing

The pacing rate is governed by several principles. First, the number of pacing stimuli per minute must always *exceed* the existing heart rate. In complete heart block, for example, where the inherent cardiac rate may be 30-40 per minute, the pacing rate would be set at 60-70 per minute. Secondly, it is undesirable to pace the heart at an overly fast rate since the oxygen demand of the myocardium is increased and patients may experience angina. Furthermore, very rapid pacing rates obviously decrease the time for ventricular filling and the cardiac output can be adversely affected in this way. Therefore, the pacing rate must be adjusted for each patient so that optimal pumping efficiency is obtained at the same time the underlying arrhythmia is being controlled.

The Energy of Pacing

In determining the energy or intensity of the stimulus required for cardiac pacing it is necessary to consider a fundamental characteristic of myocardial contractility: when the heart is stimulated by an electrical impulse it responds (contracts) either completely or not at all (the "all-or-none" law). The *lowest* electrical energy that will cause myocardial contraction is called the *threshold level.* If the intensity of a pacing stimulus is less than the threshold level contraction will *not* occur. Conversely, a pacing stimulus *greater* than the threshold level will not produce a stronger contraction, since the muscle already contracts to its fullest extent at the threshold point. In other words, there is a critical level of electrical energy below which contraction will not occur and above which it is not augmented.

Therefore in setting the intensity of the pacing impulse it is necessary to first determine the threshold level. This is accomplished as follows: after the catheter has been positioned correctly and attached to the pacemaker, the energy control dial is increased gradually from the lowest milliampere setting to a point where a QRS complex is noted with each stimulus. This setting is the threshold level.

When a catheter electrode is properly positioned and the electrode is in good contact with the endocardium, the threshold level is usually less than 2 milliamperes in most patients. If the threshold is much higher, for example 6 or 8 milliamperes, it is likely that the catheter is poorly situated in the ventricle and that repositioning of the tip is required. Because the threshold is not constant at all times and varies with the contact of the electrode tip and the endocardium, it is customary to set the energy level for pacing at twice the threshold value to overcome this variation. For example, if the threshold is found to be 1 milliampere, the final setting for the pacing stimulus should be 2 milliamperes.

Duration of Pacing

As already noted, transvenous pacing is employed fundamentally as a prophylactic measure when advanced forms of heart block or bradyarrhythmias (refractory to drugs) exist. Because these particular arrhythmic disturbances are almost always of a *transient* nature in acute myocardial infarction cardiac pacing is required only on a temporary basis until a normal rate and rhythm have returned. While the exact duration of these rhythm disturbances varied with the site of infarction and the rate of healing among other factors, most of these disorders last less than ten days and pacing is seldom required beyond this period. After normal sinus rhythm has returned it is customary to leave the pacing catheter in place for another week in the event the arrhythmia returns. Following this additional period the pacing catheter is removed.

Problems With Temperorary Transvenous Pacing

Several difficulties may be encountered during the course of temporary pacing. The most common of these are:

Displacement of the Catheter Tip

For pacing to be effective the catheter electrode must remain in proximity to the inner wall of the right ventricle. Displacement of the tip is a frequent event during temporary pacing and is undoubtedly the most common reason for pacing failure. Such displacement occurs with greater frequency when the catheter has been introduced via an arm vein (motion of the arm tends to move the entire catheter) but dislodgement of the tip may result from change of body position regardless of the insertion site.

Displacement of the pacing electrode can be suspected when each pacing stimulus fails to produce a QRS complex. This means that the pacing impulse is ineffective and is not capturing the heart beat. This *loss of capture* is shown in the following electrocardiogram. Once displacement has occurred the catheter usually has to be repositioned in the ventricle to achieve effective pacing but occasionally changing the

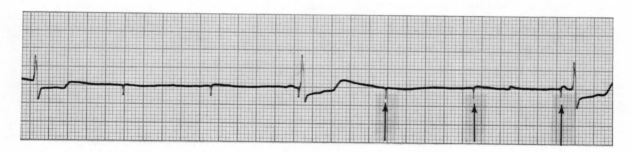

Fig. 15-12

position of the patient in bed will restore the catheter to its proper position.

The Development of Competition

As discussed previously competition of rhythms can be expected when *fixed* rate pacemakers are used. The problem is particularly common when an underlying heart block subsides and a faster normal rhythm returns. In this circumstance the natural and paced rhythms (which may be of similar rates) compete with each other. Although competition theoretically should not develop during demand pacing the problem does occur. Usually this results from inadequate sensing of the intracavitary electrocardiogram by the pacemaker. Unless the R wave returning to the sensing mechanism is of sufficient height the pacemaker will not recognize the beat and will fire an impulse; this causes competition. In this event the catheter tip must be moved to a different location in the right ventricle to obtain a better R wave signal for the sensing mechanism.

Loss of Pacing Artifact

If the pacing stimulus does not produce an artifact on the electrocardiogram it can be presumed that one of the components of the pacing system has failed. The particular problem is usually not difficult to identify. If the pulse indicator (on the face of the pacemaker) shows no impulse it implies that either the batteries are exhausted or that the pulse generator is broken. When the pacemaker is functioning, according to the pulse indicator dial, it can be reasoned that the impulse, while originating normally is not reaching the heart, either because of a broken wire within the catheter, or more simply because the catheter terminal is disconnected from the pulse generator.

Perforation of the Ventricular Wall by the Catheter Tip

Since the catheter electrode is deliberately placed against the inner surface of the ventricular wall it is understandable that the catheter tip may embed itself in the myocardium, particularly when the catheter remains in the heart for many days. In some patients the catheter actually burrows through the full thickness of the myocardium and finally perforates the right ventricular wall. This untoward event produces surprisingly few effects. Since the blood pressure within the right ventricle is normally quite low (unlike the high pressure within the left ventricle), perforation of this chamber seldom produces any hemodynamic consequences. If bleeding occurs into the pericardium it is generally trivial in amount, and does not produce cardiac tamponade.

That perforation has occurred can be suspected by a sudden loss of capture after a period of successful pacing. On some occasions the catheter perforation is recognized by the appearance of diaphragmatic or chest wall contractions. This muscle twitching, which is usually obvious to the patient, signifies that the catheter electrode has perforated the right ventricle and has travelled to the diaphragm or intercostal muscles. This diagnosis can often be confirmed by means of a chest x-ray which shows the catheter tip outside the right ventricle.

When perforation of the ventricle occurs it is necessary to withdraw the catheter and resposition it in the right ventricle.

Thrombophlebitis and Skin Infections

Since catheters must often remain in the venous system for prolonged periods there is always the possibility that thrombophlebitis may develop from mechanical irritation of the vein wall. The likelihood of this inflammatory reaction is perhaps increased when smaller veins are used as insertion sites (e.g., arm veins), however other factors undoubtedly contribute to this complication. If thrombophlebitis is marked the catheter must be removed and another one inserted in a different vein.Because the skin puncture site is, in effect, an open wound, local infection in this area may occur. This risk can be minimized (almost excluded) by adherence to strict surgical asepsis at the time of catheter placement and by the use of antibiotic (neomycin) ointment subsequently.

The Nursing Role in Cardiac Pacing

Preparation For Catheter Insertion

1) When a decision has been made to pace the heart temporarily it is important to explain to the patient why the procedure is necessary and how it is performed. The emphasis of the explanation should be on the preventive benefit derived from controlling the heart rate with pacing.

2) If cardiac pacing is to be performed on an *elective* basis (e.g., a patient with second degree heart block) it is customary to have an operative permit signed by the patient. Obviously in emergency situations this measure can be disregarded.

3) If the catheter is to be positioned by electrocardiographic rather than fluoroscopic means, the limb lead electrodes should be attached to all of the extremities and a separate ECG machine prepared for use. After the catheter has been inserted into the venous system, the chest (V) lead terminal is then connected to the free end of the pacing catheter by means of an "alligator" clamp to record the intracavitary tracing (which identifies the position of the catheter electrode). It is essential that *all* of the equipment used be grounded properly to prevent the threat of electrocution by extraneous electrical current passing through the catheter *to* the heart. Some institutions use battery powered electrocardiographic machines to obviate this problem.

4) A syringe containing 100 mg. of lidocaine should be prepared and placed at the bedside. In addition, the nurse should verify the patency of the pre-existing "keep-open" intravenous line. This preparedness is essential to combat any ventricular irritability that may develop suddenly during manipulation of the catheter within the heart.

5) A defibrillator should be available for immediate use in the event (even though unlikely) that the catheter may induce ventricular fibrillation.

Catheter Insertion

1) The skin surrounding the intended site of catheter insertion is prepared with soap, alcohol, and a skin antiseptic, as customary with any surgical procedure. An "eye sheet" is used to drape the area leaving only the operative site exposed. In addition, the patient's face is covered with a loose

drape to prevent breath contamination. (Pathogens from the mouth and nose are a far greater source of wound infection than bacteria found on the skin.)

2) The needle placement set and the appropriate catheter should be sterile and ready for use. Sterilization can be accomplished by the use of bacteriocidal solutions or by gas techniques; autoclaving should not be used because of the plastic materials contained in the catheter and in the needle sheath.

3) A local anesthetic (procaine or lidocaine) is used to infiltrate the skin before the large-bore needle is inserted into the vein.

4) As the catheter is advanced into the heart the electrocardiogram must be monitored with great care to detect premature ventricular beats that may develop. This means the electrocardiogram must be observed *continuously* during the procedure, either with a customary monitoring system (or with a separate ECG machine if placement is guided by an intracavitary electrode).

5) After the physician has placed the catheter in proper position and effective capture of the heart beat is achieved, the catheter must be secured. This may be accomplished by placing a suture around the catheter and through the skin, or more simply, by adhesive tapes. An antibiotic ointment (neomycin or bacitracin) is then applied to the skin entry site and a dry dressing is firmly affixed.

Subsequent Care

The major responsibility of the nurse during the course of cardiac pacing is to verify that the pacemaker system is functioning properly and effectively.

As noted, there are several problems which may arise during temporary pacing and careful observation of the patient and the monitor is essential to detect these disturbances as soon as they occur:

1) If there is loss of capture (as noted in the following rhythm strip) the nurse should notify the physician immediately because the pacing stimulus is wholly ineffective in this situation. Depending on the underlying arrhythmias for which pacing is being used, loss of capture can be associated with serious consequences. For example, if pacing fails during complete heart block, ventricular standstill may result. (Fig. 15-13).

2) A second situation demanding emergency action is the sudden disappearance of pacing artifacts on the electrocardiogram. (Fig. 15-14). On many occasions the cause of this crisis can be instantly identified and corrected by the nurse. The first step in solving the problem is to make

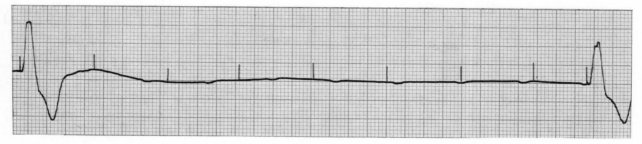

Fig. 15-13

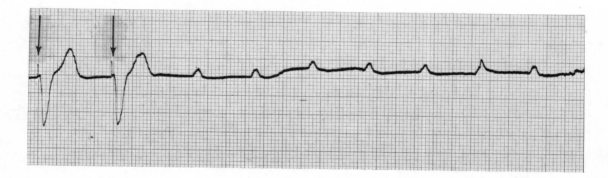

Fig. 15-14

certain the catheter terminals have not become disconnected from the pacemaker device. If these connections are secure the next thing to do is to ascertain that an adequate stimulus is being generated by the battery. If there is no movement of the pulse indicator, the pacemaker batteries may be exhausted and the pacemaker should be replaced. (To prevent this latter catastrophe a careful record should be kept of the number of hours each pacemaker is actually used. While the effective battery life of most pulse generators is presumably 800 hours, it is a good practice to routinely change batteries after 600 hours of use.) If the problem cannot be corrected instantly (as in the example shown above), cardiopulmonary resuscitation should be initiated without delay.

3) Of less urgent importance than loss of capture or pacemaker failure is the development of competition between the paced and natural cardiac rhythms. If competition occurs during fixed rate pacing it may indicate that normal sinus rhythm has returned. The presence of competition during demand pacing suggests difficulty with the sensing system of the pacemaker unit. In either instance the nurse should apprise the physician of this undesirable rhythm.

4) The sudden appearance of diaphragmatic or chest wall contractions, synchronous with pacing impulses, should be cause for suspicion that the catheter tip has perforated the right ventricular wall.The nurse should report this complication to the physician immediately.

5) The nurse should carefully examine the catheter insertion site twice a day for signs of local infection. Antibiotic ointment should be applied daily. In addition, signs of thrombophlebitis should be sought, particularly when the catheter has been introduced by way of an arm vein.

PRECORDIAL SHOCK

The Concept of Precordial Shock

Precordial shock is used as a life-saving emergency method for terminating ventricular fibrillation (defibrillation), as well as an elective procedure to convert certain atrial and ventricular tachyarrhythmias (cardioversion) to normal rhythm.

The principle of precordial shock in treating ventricular fibrillation is not complicated: a high voltage shock of very brief duration (only a few thousandths of one second) delivered through the chest wall is capable of abruptly stopping the chaotic electrical activity within the heart that produced this lethal arrhythmia. Once the bizarre fibrillatory rhythm is terminated in this way, the heart's natural pacemaker regains command and an effective beat is re-established.

This same principle is also utilized in elective cardioversion where brief depolarization of the entire heart (at a particular time in the cardiac cycle) halts the ectopic pacemaker and allows the SA node to again assume control.

While enormous electrical energy (about 7000 volts) are required to depolarize the heart through the chest wall, this electrical force is so very short in duration that the current does not injure the heart.

The Equipment

Precordial shock to terminate ventricular fibrillation can be delivered by means of either an alternating current (AC) or a direct current (DC) defibrillator. While both types of defibrillators are equally effective for this purpose the direct current defibrillator can also be used for elective precordial shock and because of this greater versatility, DC machines are used almost routinely in coronary care units.

The direct current defibrillator builds and stores thousands of volts in a capacitor, within seconds, and discharges this energy, on demand, in less than 10 milliseconds. The stored energy is discharged by pressing a switch located either on the machine itself, or on the handles of the paddle electrodes. Foot switches are also available but these are not desirable because of the risk of inadvertently stepping on them during the confusion of an emergency and accidently discharging the defibrillator. The amount of energy to be delivered by the defibrillator can be controlled with a dial setting. This electrical force is calculated in terms of *watt-seconds*; the scale usually ranges from 1-400 watt-seconds.

The electrodes, or paddles as they are called, which are held against the chest wall have insulated handles to protect the operator. These paddles are large (generally 3-4 inches in diameter) allowing the electrical discharge to be delivered over a large skin area in order to prevent electrical burns. A thick layer of conductive paste is applied to skin and electrode surfaces before the energy is discharged.

Synchronized and Non-synchronized Precordial Shock

When precordial shock is used to convert atrial and ventricular tachyarrhythmias (cardioversion), it is important that the electrical discharge be synchronized with the cardiac cycle. This need can be appreciated on the following basis: when an electrical impulse, even a premature ventricular contraction, strikes during the vulnerable period of the cardiac cycle (that is, during the time of T wave as shown in (Fig. 15-15) there is a potential danger of inducing *ventricular fibrillation*. The same

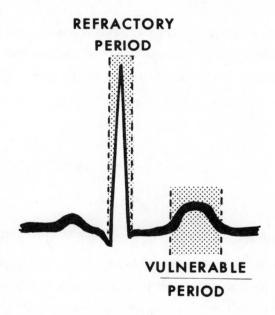

REFRACTORY
PERIOD

VULNERABLE
PERIOD

Fig. 15-15

threat may exist if a precordial shock (or a pacemaker impulse) arrives during this critical interval. To avoid this hazard precordial shock is deliberately *synchronized* so that the electrical force is delivered at a point in the cardiac cycle when the heart is *refractory* to stimulation; this *non-vulnerable* period exists during the time of the QRS complex. The equipment is so designed that the discharge energy can be synchronized with the safe (the refractory) period of the cardiac cycle. When the synchronizer switch is *on* and the discharge button is triggered, the instrument waits until the next R wave before delivering its energy. On the other hand, if the synchronizer is *off*, discharge occurs at the instant the machine is triggered without reference to the cardiac cycle.

It is essential to clearly understand just when precordial shock should, or should not, be synchronized. *In terminating ventricular fibrillation with precordial shock (defibrillation), the synchronizer switch must be in the OFF position.* If the synchronizer switch is *on* in this circumstance, the machine will *not* fire in that it awaits a QRS complex which, of course, is non-existent during ventricular fibrillation.

Conversely, when precordial shock is employed *electively* to convert other arrhythmias (e.g., atrial fibrillation) the synchronizer must be *ON* to avoid the possibility of the discharge striking during the vulnerable period and inducing ventricular fibrillation.

The Energy of Discharge

As indicated, the level of discharge energy is adjustable and must be set for the particular arrhythmias being treated. *For ventricular fibrillation the maximum energy (400 watt-seconds) should always be used.* With elective cardioversion, the precise energy setting varies with several factors — the most important of which are the particular arrhythmia being treated, and whether the patient is receiving digitalis concomitantly. Many physicians prefer to attempt cardioversion using very low energies (e.g., 25 watt seconds or less) at first and if the trial is unsuccessful to increase the levels on successive attempts until conversion is achieved; others use higher energies (e.g., 200 watt seconds or more) initially.

The Technique of Elective Cardioversion and the Nursing Role

Preparation for Procedure

1) The procedure should be explained to the patient by a member of the nurse-physician team. Because the word "shock" has frightening connotations, it is wise to avoid using this term in describing the treatment.

2) It is customary, in many institutions, to have an operative permit signed by the patient when an elective cardioversion is to be performed.

3) All necessary equipment and materials should be at the bedside. This includes the machine which delivers the synchronized shock, along with syringes, antiarrhythmic drugs, and anesthetic agents.

4) Although elective cardioversion is a remarkably safe procedure when properly performed the theoretical possibility exists that the shock might induce ventricular fibrillation. For this reason, emergency equipment for cardiopulmonary resuscitation, (e.g., a manual breathing bag, airways, etc.) should be in readiness. A syringe containing 100 mg. of lidocaine should always be at the bedside for immediate use.

5) An intravenous pathway must be established and its patency verified, prior to the procedure. This conduit is used to administer the anesthetic agent and antiarrhythmic drugs that may be necessary.

6) The skin electrodes from the cardioversion equipment are attached to the patient so that the electrical shock can be synchronized with the R wave of the cardiac cycle. (With some machines the customary monitoring electrodes can be used for this purpose and these additional electrodes are unnecessary.)

Setting the Machine For Cardioversion

1) The synchronizer switch is turned ON so that the discharge of energy will coincide with the R wave of the cardiac cycle.

2) Because synchronization cannot be achieved unless the ventricular complexes are of sufficient amplitude to trigger the discharge, the "gain," dial may have to be adjusted to obtain R waves of adequate size (as evidenced by a flashing light or other signal). If complexes of sufficient height cannot be obtained by increasing the gain, a different lead must be used to achieve taller waves. (e.g., changing from Lead II to Lead I).

3) With some equipment the discharge can be synchronized with deep S waves as well as tall R waves. When the S wave is used for this purpose the polarity switch, which is kept in the positive (+) position for R wave synchronization, must be changed to the negative (−) side.

4) For safety, it is wise to verify that proper synchronization will occur when the machine is fired. This is accomplished by a test mechanism within the machine which indicates where the discharge will fall in the cardiac cycle when the shock is actually delivered.

5) The energy (watt-seconds) to be used for the cardioversion attempt is set at the desired level by the physician.

Anesthesia

Although precordial shock itself creates little actual pain because of the extremely short duration of the stimulus, the sensation (and the associated generalized muscle contraction) is nevertheless frightening and unpleasant for most patients. For this reason it is customary to use general anesthesia for the procedure. Because an analgesic effect is required for only a few seconds, very short acting agents, such as sodium methohexital (Brevital) or diazepam (Valium), are given intravenously just before the shock is delivered.

Paddle Electrodes: Preparation and Placement

1) Prior to the procedure paddles should be carefully cleaned with scouring powder to remove metallic oxides which form on the surface of the electrodes and interfere with the flow of current.

2) A thick layer of conducting jelly is placed on the face of the electrodes and distributed evenly. Additional electrode paste is applied to the chest wall where the paddles will be held. Unless there is an adequate amount of jelly at the electrode-skin interface, serious skin burns can occur.

3) One paddle is placed in the right sternal area and the other on the left lateral chest wall. The precise location of the paddles is not critical as long as the flow of current traverses the heart. (See Fig. 15-16)

An alternative method of paddle placement is to position one electrode (a special flat paddle) under the left scapula and to hold the other paddle directly over the upper sternum (see Fig. 15-17). In this way the flow of current passes directly through the heart in an anterior-posterior direction.

4) Before the energy is discharged it is important to ascertain that the conducting paste remains localized at the electrode sites and has not spread over the chest wall. Excess jelly should be wiped dry before proceeding or else the current will flow across the skin surface (rather than through the heart) creating a large spark.

5) The paddles are pressed firmly and evenly against the chest wall; failure to preserve good contact results in dissipation of energy. Furthermore, tilting of the paddles may cause skin burns.

6) Since there is a theoretical threat that the electrical force being delivered to the patient could pass through the bed and reach the operator it is a wise practice to have all personnel stand clear at the moment of discharge.

7) The discharge switch is pressed and the effect is immediately evident by a sudden generalized contraction of the patient's muscles. Observation of the oscilloscope will confirm whether normal rhythm has been restored.

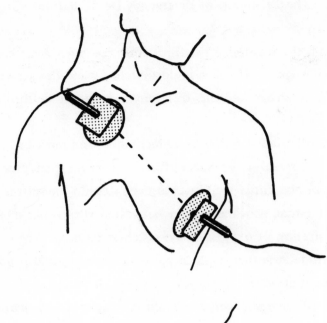

Fig. 15-16

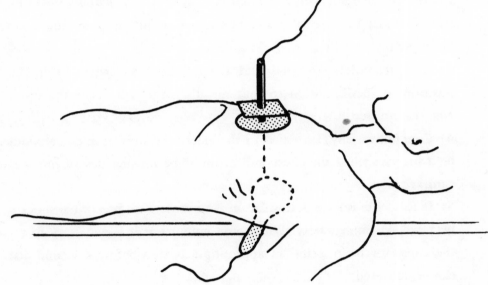

Fig. 15-17

8) In some instances, premature ventricular contractions are noted following cardioversion and lidocaine should be administered promptly to combat this cardiac irritability.

9) In the extremely unlikely event that the cardioversion attempt causes ventricular fibrillation the synchronizer switch must be turned OFF, the energy increased to 400 watt seconds, and a second shock delivered instantly to defibrillate the patient. Remember that defibrillation cannot be accomplished if the synchronizer is on!

The Technique of Emergency Defibrillation

Although the method for defibrillation has been described in the discussion of ventricular fibrillation (page 175), it is important to review this procedure in additional detail with particular emphasis on the differences between defibrillation and elective cardioversion.

1) Defibrillation is a life-saving technique, and must be accomplished within a minute or so to be successful. This means that precordial shock must always be the *initial* step in treatment (within the setting of a coronary care unit) and that no time should be wasted with other measures, such as the administration of oxygen or closed chest massage. The first person reaching the bedside, whether a physician or a nurse, should proceed to defibrillate the patient at once.

2) The discharge energy should be set at its *maximum* level: 400 watt-seconds; the use of lesser energies is pointless and should never be attempted.

3) It is absolutely essential that the synchronizer switch be in the OFF position for defibrillation so that the discharge will occur the instant the trigger is pressed.

4) Conductive jelly is applied to the electrode surfaces and the paddles are held firmly against the chest wall in the same manner described for elective cardioversion.

5) If for some reason defibrillation is unsuccessful, precordial shock should be repeated immediately. With some equipment it is necessary to recharge the capacitor by pressing an appropriate button before a second discharge can be delivered.

EXERCISES IN THE
INTERPRETATION OF ARRHYTHMIAS

On the following pages, 30 electrocardiographic rhythm strips are presented for interpretation.

This exercise is meant to serve several purposes:

a) to permit self-testing of the ability to identify common arrhythmias

b) to demonstrate variations in the patterns of certain arrhythmias

c) to introduce a few less-common arrhythmias not described in previous chapters.

Interpretations of these electrocardiograms along with pertinent comments are found on the back of each page.

It is important to realize that many arrhythmias <u>cannot</u> be identified with certainty from a single rhythm strip and that multiple leads are often necessary to reach a definite conclusion. When doubt exists, it is a wise practice to state that there are one or more possibilities in interpretation (e.g., the arrhythmia may be <u>either</u> sinus tachycardia <u>or</u> atrial tachycardia).

EXAMPLES

ECG #1

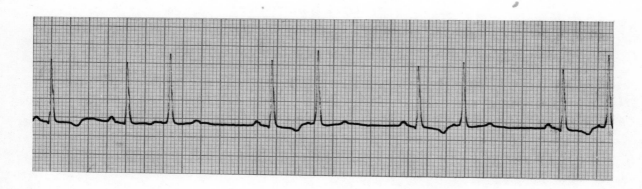

ECG #2

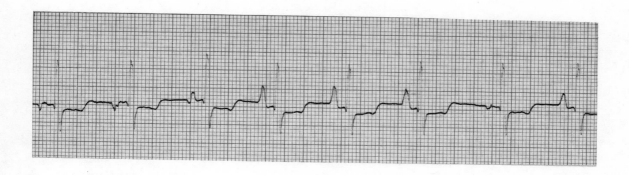

ECG #3

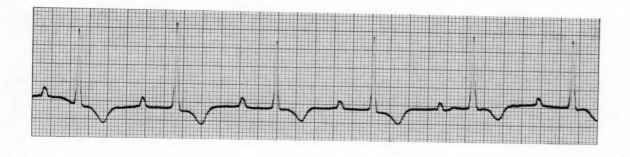

Example #1

Premature Atrial Contractions

Every <u>second</u> beat is a premature atrial contraction. This pattern is described as <u>atrial bigeminy</u>. That the ectopic beats are atrial in origin is apparent from the contour of the P waves which differ distinctly from those associated with the normal beats originating in the SA node.

Example #2

Wandering Pacemaker

The P waves have different configurations with some being inverted and the others upright. This indicates that the pacemaker wanders between the AV node (the first two complexes) and the SA node.

Example #3

First Degree AV Block

The P-R interval measures .36 seconds. This prolongation (greater than .20 seconds) is diagnostic of first degree AV heart block. The inverted T waves reflect myocardial ischemia.

ECG #4

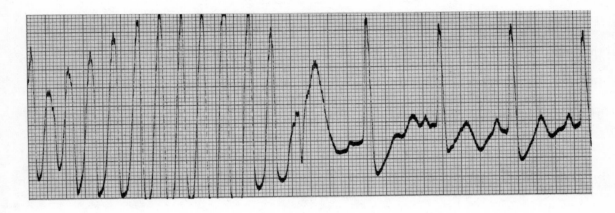

ECG #5

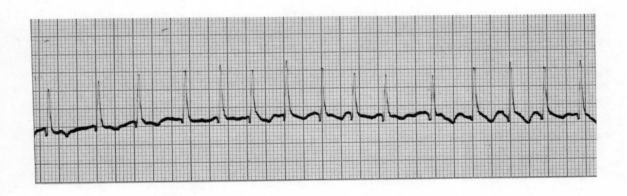

ECG #6

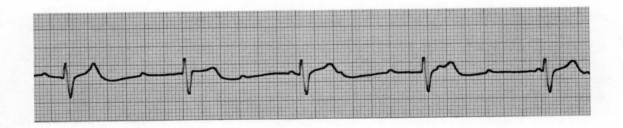

INTERPRETATION OF ELECTROCARDIOGRAMS

Example #4

Extreme Ventricular Tachycardia (Ventricular Flutter)

Returning to Normal Sinus Rhythm

The initial complexes which occur at a rate of more than 200 per minute show the typical helix-like pattern of extreme ventricular tachycardia (ventricular flutter). This arrhythmia was treated with 100 mg. of lidocaine intravenously after which sinus rhythm was restored as noted in the last complexes. If lidocaine fails to terminate ventricular flutter immediately, precordial shock should be used without delay.

Example #5

Atrial Fibrillation

The obvious irregularity of the R-R intervals along with the absence of P waves is characteristic of atrial fibrillation. The rapid ventricular response (rate about 150 per minute) indicates that the atrial fibrillation is uncontrolled. Fibrillatory waves ('f' waves) are interspersed and occasionally appear to mimic P waves, but the irregularity of these waves excludes this latter possibility.

Example #6

Third Degree (Complete AV Heart Block)

The P waves bear no relationship to the QRS complexes and the atrial and ventricular pacemakers are independent (AV dissociation). The atrial rate is about 120 per minute and the ventricular rate is 47 per minute. The ventricular rate represents the inherent discharge rate of the ventricles and in most instances is less than 40 per minute although rates up to 50 per minute can exist (as in this example).

ECG #7

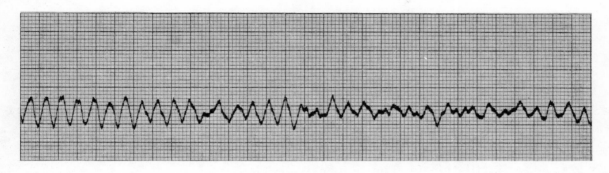

ECG #8

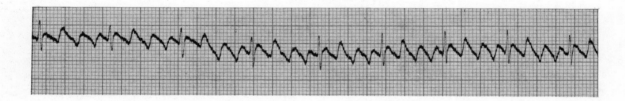

ECG #9

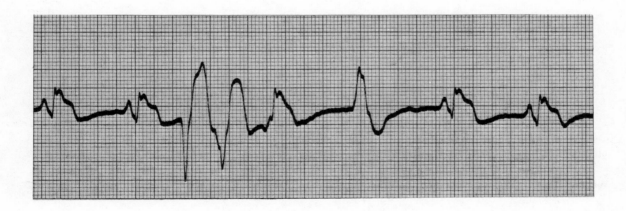

Example #7

Ventricular Fibrillation

The bizarre, chaotic waves are characteristic of ventricular fibrillation. The initial complexes seem to have a certain regularity and demonstrate the pre-fibrillatory pattern which is transitional between ventricular flutter and ventricular fibrillation. This intimate relationship between ventricular flutter and ventricular fibrillation is thus demonstrated here.

Example #8

Atrial Flutter With 4:1 Block

The atrial rate is 320 per minute while the ventricular rate is 80 per minute. The P waves have been replaced by typical flutter waves ("F" waves) creating the classical "saw-tooth" configuration of atrial flutter.

Example #9

Multifocal Premature Ventricular Contractions

The ectopic ventricular beats are widened and distorted in shape and arise from different foci in the ventricles as evidenced by their varying configurations. The remaining complexes, originating in the SA node, show deep Q waves and marked elevation of the S-T segments. This combination (Q waves and S-T segment elevation) is typical of acute myocardial infarction.

ECG #10

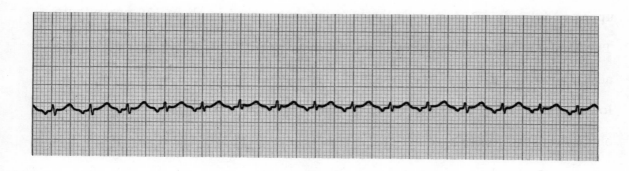

ECG #11

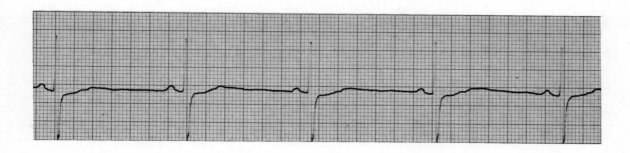

ECG #12

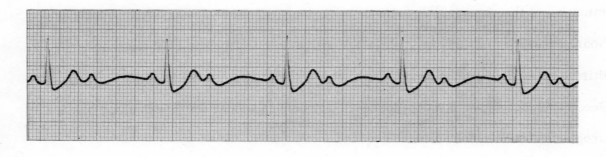

INTERPRETATION OF ELECTROCARDIOGRAMS

Example #10

Paroxysmal Nodal Tachycardia

The P waves are <u>inverted</u> and <u>precede</u> the QRS complexes. This indicates an upper nodal origin of the arrhythmia. The heart rate is about 150 per minute. The low amplitude of the complexes as recorded with the monitor lead is disadvantageous and makes the interpretation more difficult. This problem of low amplitude may be resolved by changing the position of the electrodes to obtain a different lead.

Example #11

Sinus Bradycardia

The primary abnormality is the slow heart rate (45 per minute). The presence of normal P waves preceding the QRS complexes indicate that the arrhythmia originated in the SA node and excludes the possibility that the slow rate is due to either a nodal rhythm or heart block. The use of atropine will usually increase the slow rate of sinus bradycardia.

Example #12

Second Degree AV Heart Block

There are <u>two</u> P waves for each QRS complex, with the atrial rate being 96 per minute and the ventricular rate 48 per minute. The P waves occur evenly and bear a direct relationship to the QRS complexes unlike the circumstances of third degree (complete) heart block where the P-R interval is totally inconstant. Second degree block is considered an advanced form of AV heart block and may progress to complete block.

ECG #13

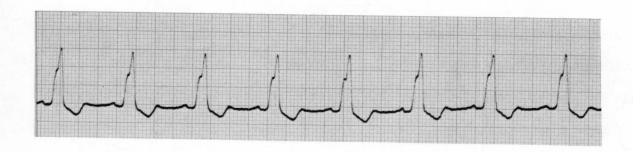

ECG #14

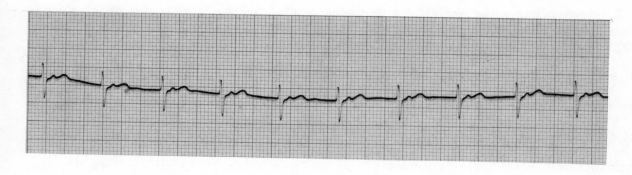

ECG #15

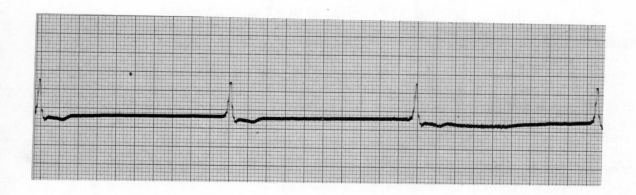

INTERPRETATION OF ELECTROCARDIOGRAMS

Example #13

Bundle Branch Block (intraventricular conduction defect)

The duration of the QRS complex is .14 seconds. This prolongation (greater than .10 seconds) indicates a defect in conduction from the AV node to the ventricular muscle. From this single monitor lead it is not possible to ascertain whether the left or right bundle branch is blocked; a full 12 lead electrocardiogram is necessary for this purpose.

Example #14

Nodal Rhythm

The P waves occur after the QRS complexes. This indicates that the pacemaker is in the lower AV node. When the AV node serves as the pacemaker its inherent rate is from 40 to 60 per minute. In this case, the rate is 96 per minute. Because of this faster than anticipated rate, this nodal rhythm must be considered as nodal tachycardia of a non-paroxysmal type. It differs from paroxysmal nodal tachycardia where the rate is greater than 100 per minute. Nodal rhythms are also described as "junctional" rhythms because of their anatomical origin in the AV node.

Example #15

Atrial Standstill With Nodal (Functional) Rhythm

The absence of P waves and the essentially straight lines between QRS complexes indicate that the SA node (or other atrial sites) no longer function as pacemakers and that atrial standstill exists. The ventricular rate is about 30 per minute. The QRS complexes are essentially normal. These latter facts imply that the AV node has assumed the pacemaking function. Were the QRS complexes widened and distorted it could be assumed that the pacemaker had descended to the ventricles rather than the AV node.

ECG #16

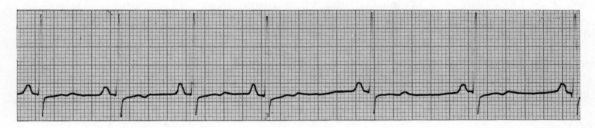

ECG #17

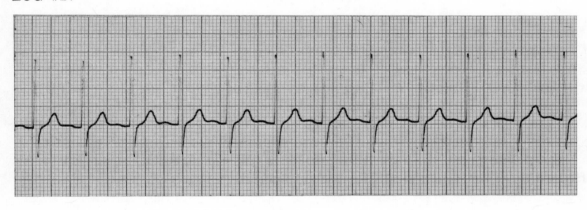

ECG #18

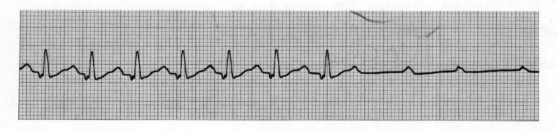

INTERPRETATION OF ELECTROCARDIOGRAMS

Example #16

Sinus Arrhythmia

The R-R intervals are irregular and vary more than .12 seconds. Because each QRS complex is preceded by a normal P wave it can be concluded that the irregular rhythm is the result of an unevenness in the rate of SA node discharges. This variation is caused by a changing vagal influence on the SA node.

Example #17

Sinus Tachycardia

The heart rate is about 120 per minute. To distinguish the exact site of this tachycardia (i.e., sinus, atrial, or nodal tachycardia) it is essential to identify P waves. In this tracing the P waves are of low amplitude and somewhat difficult to see without scrutiny. This problem can be clarified by choosing a different lead for monitoring which shows the P waves more clearly.

Example #18

Primary Ventricular Standstill

The QRS complexes cease abruptly, while P wave activity continues. This means that ventricular activation has stopped (i.e., ventricular standstill). This sudden loss of ventricular function results in circulatory arrest as evidenced by unconsciousness and the absence of heart sounds and peripheral pulses. The catastrophe is described as a Stokes-Adams attack. Unless ventricular function is restored within a minute or so, death will follow.

ECG #19

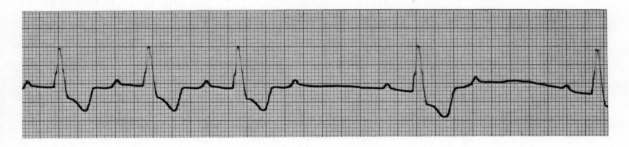

ECG #20

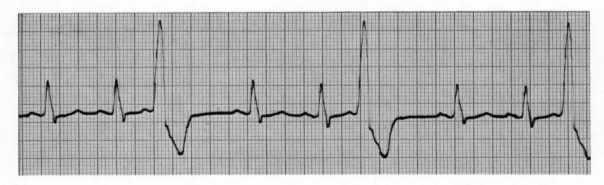

ECG #21

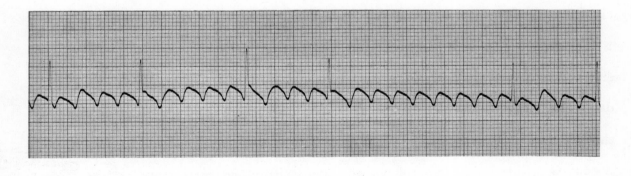

INTERPRETATION OF ELECTROCARDIOGRAMS

Example #19

The Development of Second Degree AV Block Following First Degree AV Block

The initial complexes show a first degree heart block (the P-R interval measures .36 seconds) with each P wave followed by a QRS complex. After the third complex, only every _other_ P wave is followed by a QRS complex (i.e., second degree heart block). This sequence differs from the Wenckebach Phenomenon in which the P-R interval lengthens progressively with successive beats until one QRS complex is dropped. The widened QRS complexes (.12 seconds) indicate that an intraventricular conduction defect is also present.

Example #20

Frequent Premature Ventricular Contractions (Trigeminy)

Every _third_ complex is a premature ventricular contraction. This sequence of two normal beats and one premature ventricular contraction is described as _trigeminy_. (When every _second_ beat is a premature ventricular contraction, the pattern is termed _bigeminy_.) Because the premature ventricular contractions all have the same configuration it can be assumed that they arose from one irritable focus (unifocal rather than multifocal origin) within the ventricle.

Example #21

Atrial Flutter with Varying Degree of Block

The presence of atrial flutter is readily identified by the occurrence of regular flutter waves ("F" waves) and the "saw-tooth" appearance they produce. The degree of block in the AV node is _inconstant_ as noted by the irregular rhythm of the QRS complexes and the varying number of F waves between complexes. Varying block of this type is common with atrial flutter and sometimes reflects overdosage of digitalis.

ECG #22

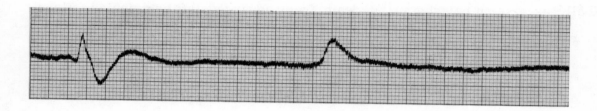

ECG #23

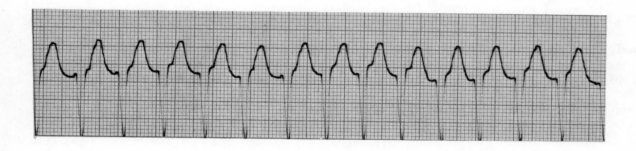

ECG #24

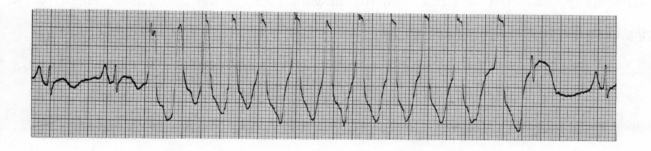

INTERPRETATION OF ELECTROCARDIOGRAMS

Example #22
Secondary Ventricular Standstill (Dying Heart Pattern)

Although there are occasional periods of electrical activity within the ventricle, these are meaningless and do not result in ventricular contraction. This isolated activity is found typically as a terminal rhythm at death from advanced left ventricular failure (secondary ventricular standstill).

Example #23
Supraventricular Tachycardia

From this single lead it is difficult to classify this arrhythmia in any more specific terms than "supraventricular tachycardia." In other words, it cannot be stated with certainty whether this arrhythmia is paroxysmal atrial tachycardia, nodal tachycardia or even sinus tachycardia and the general classification of supraventricular tachycardia is used. The obstacle in interpretation relates to the inability to distinguish P waves from this monitor lead. That the arrhythmia may be ventricular tachycardia is unlikely because of the normal duration of the QRS complexes.

Example #24
Paroxysmal Ventricular Tachycardia

After two normally conducted beats from the SA node, a premature ventricular beat occurs. This ectopic beat strikes during the upstroke of the inverted T wave of the last normally conducted beat (i.e., during the vulnerable phase) and causes repetitive firing of the irritable ventricular focus. This results in a consecutive series of premature ventricular contractions. By definition this sequence of four or more consecutive PVCs represents ventricular tachycardia. This episode of ventricular tachycardia stopped spontaneously; however, sustained ventricular tachycardia could also have occurred.

ECG #25

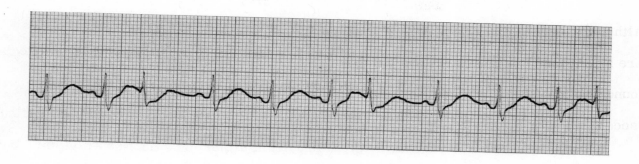

ECG #26

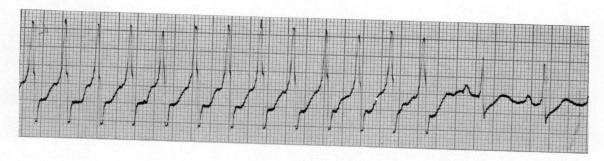

ECG #27

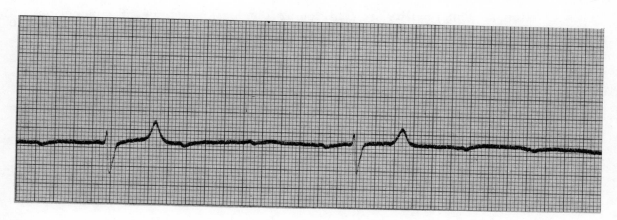

Example #25

Premature Nodal Contractions

In the presence of a normal sinus rhythm there are frequent premature nodal contractions.   The P waves of these ectopic beats are <u>inverted</u> and occur immediately <u>before</u> the QRS complexes.   Conduction from the AV node to the ventricles is normal as evidenced by the unchanged shape of the QRS complexes.   It is often difficult to distinguish premature nodal contractions from premature atrial contractions, but the presence of an inverted P wave with a P-R interval of less than .12 seconds is typical of PNCs and justifies this diagnosis.

Example #26

Supraventricular Tachycardia
(Probably Paroxysmal Atrial Tachycardia With Aberrant Conduction)

The occurrence of very rapid, regular QRS complexes (about 180 per minute) in conjunction with abnormally shaped and positioned P waves (preceding the QRS complexes) suggests this arrhythmia is paroxysmal atrial tachycardia. The abrupt cessation of the tachycardia (see last complexes) is a characteristic feature of PAT. Because of the rapidity of atrial impulses the ventricles are unable to recover (repolarize) fully from the previous contraction before the next impulse arrives. This creates an abnormality in ventricular conduction (aberrant conduction) which affects the shape of the QRS complexes.

Example #27

Complete Heart Block Leading To Ventricular Standstill

During the course of complete heart block, the ventricular pacemaker failed gradually. The heart rate is only 20 per minute and the QRS complexes occur irregularly. In effect, ventricular standstill has developed. The patient died within minutes after this electrocardiogram was obtained.

ECG #28

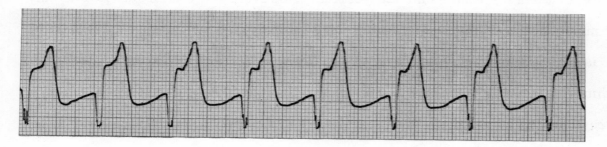

ECG #29

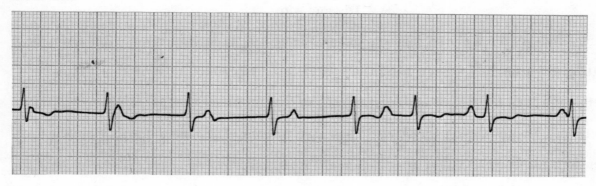

ECG #30

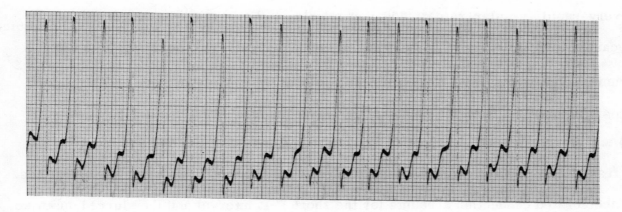

INTERPRETATION OF ELECTROCARDIOGRAMS

Example #28
"Slow" Ventricular Tachycardia or Idioventricular Rhythm

This series of eight consecutive premature ventricular contractions would fulfill the diagnostic criteria for ventricular tachycardia. However, the ventricular rate is only 80 per minute and actually cannot be considered a tachycardia. Because of this latter fact it is difficult to properly classify this arrhythmia. Many clinicians describe this arrhythmia as "slow" ventricular tachycardia while others choose the term idioventricular rhythm (implying simply that the arrhythmia arises in the ventricle). This semantic problem has yet to be settled.

Example #29
AV Dissociation

The atria and ventricles are beating independently of each other with the SA node controlling the atria and the AV node the ventricles. Because the rhythms are dissociated the P waves bear no fixed relationship to the QRS complexes. This arrhythmia differs from complete heart block (which is also a form of AV dissociation) in that the ventricular rate is equal to (or greater than) the atrial rate.

Example #30
Paroxysmal Atrial Tachycardia Due To The Wolff-Parkinson-White Syndrome

The very rapid, regular rate of 200 per minute is the result of paroxysmal atrial tachycardia. The etiology of this episode of atrial tachycardia differs from the usual mechanism and is due to the Wolff-Parkinson-White (W-P-W) syndrome. This latter diagnosis is apparent from the combination of very short P-R intervals (about .08 seconds) and slurred widened QRS complexes. It is believed that the impulse from the SA node traverses a shorter-than-normal (an accessory) pathway in reaching the ventricles. This accelerated conduction accounts for the short P-R interval and the slurred upstroke of the R wave. Paroxysmal atrial tachycardia is a common event among patients with W-P-W syndrome.

Index